100 Uplifting Short Stories for Elderly

MARIA VAN KOUCHY

Table of Contents

How Sweet Surprises Can Bring Joy to Life's Journey"

The morning sun shone bright and golden, casting its warm rays on the sleepy town of Belleview. The bustling streets were alive with the sound of birds chirping and people chattering away, enjoying the beginning of a new day. One such person was Miss Lucy, an elderly lady who had lived in Belleview all her life.

Miss Lucy was a cheerful soul, with a twinkle in her eye and a spring in her step. She was known throughout the town for her sweet demeanor and kind heart. Her bright smile never failed to light up the faces of those around her. Today was no exception as she made her way to the local bakery to pick up some freshly baked bread.

As she entered the bakery, the delicious aroma of cinnamon and sugar wafted through the air, making her mouth water. She was greeted by the friendly baker, Mr. Henry, who always had a warm smile for her. After exchanging some pleasantries, Miss Lucy placed her order and began to peruse the shelves.

Suddenly, she heard a commotion outside. Curious, she made her way to the window and peered outside. To her surprise, she saw a young man, no more than twenty, standing in the middle of the street, looking lost and confused. He was holding a small bag and appeared to be searching for something.

Without thinking twice, Miss Lucy rushed out of the bakery and approached the young man. "Excuse me, dear, can I help you with something?" she asked, her kind eyes shining with concern.

The young man looked up, startled, and shook his head. "No, ma'am, I'm fine. I'm just looking for a place to stay for the night. My car broke down and I'm stranded here."

Miss Lucy's heart went out to the young man. "Well, you're in luck, dear. I have a spare room at my house, and you're more than welcome to stay with me for as long as you need."

The young man's face lit up with gratitude, and he thanked her profusely. As they made their way to Miss Lucy's house, they chatted and got to know each other better. His name was Tom, and he was a musician, traveling from town to town, playing his guitar and singing his heart out.

Over the next few days, Miss Lucy and Tom became the best of friends. He would play his guitar for her, and she would regale him with stories of her youth. They would go on walks together and explore the town, visiting old landmarks and reminiscing about times gone by.

One day, Tom surprised Miss Lucy with a gift - a freshly baked cake from the local bakery. "It's a thank you for being so kind to me," he said, his eyes twinkling.

Miss Lucy was touched by the gesture, and together, they enjoyed the delicious cake, laughing and chatting away. As they sat there, Miss Lucy felt a sense of nostalgia wash over her. She thought about her youth and the many adventures she had experienced. She looked at Tom, and realized that he reminded her of someone - a young man she had once loved, many years ago.

Tears welled up in her eyes, and Tom noticed her sadness. "What's wrong, Miss Lucy?" he asked, concerned.

Miss Lucy took a deep breath and smiled through her tears. "Oh, nothing, dear. I was just thinking about the past. It's amazing how life comes full circle. You remind me of someone I loved a long time ago."

Tom looked at her, his eyes filled with understanding. "Well, Miss Lucy, I am glad I can bring back those memories for you. I believe that everything happens for a reason, and perhaps I was meant to come into your life and remind you of the good times."

Miss Lucy smiled at Tom, feeling grateful for his company and his wise words. "You're right, dear. Life is full of surprises, and you, my young friend, are the sweetest surprise of all."

As they finished their cake and watched the sun set over the town, Miss Lucy felt a sense of contentment wash over her. She had found a new friend, and together, they would create new memories and cherish the old ones.

From that day on, Tom became a regular visitor

at Miss Lucy's house. They would spend hours chatting and laughing, and sometimes, Tom would even play his guitar and sing for her. The people of Belleview noticed how happy Miss Lucy had become, and they couldn't help but smile whenever they saw the two of them together.

Years went by, and Miss Lucy grew old, but her spirit remained as bright and cheerful as ever. Tom continued to visit her, even after he became a famous musician, traveling the world and playing in sold-out concerts. He always made time for his dear friend Miss Lucy, and she never forgot the sweetest surprise life had given her.

In the end, Miss Lucy passed away peacefully in her sleep, surrounded by the memories of a life well-lived. Tom, who had become like family to her, played a special song at her funeral, a tribute to the woman who had touched his life in so many ways.

As the townsfolk said their goodbyes and scattered flowers over her grave, they couldn't help but feel grateful for the sweetest surprise life had given them - the gift of Miss Lucy and her infectious joy.

The Lost Key

It was a sunny afternoon when Mr. and Mrs. Jenkins returned home from their grocery shopping. They had a wonderful day, but as soon as they reached their doorstep, they realized that they had lost their house key.

"Oh no, what are we going to do?" said Mrs. Jenkins.

"We could call the locksmith, but that would be expensive," replied Mr. Jenkins.

Just then, their neighbor, Mrs. Wilson, came out of her house.

"Is everything okay?" she asked.

"We lost our house key," explained Mrs. Jenkins.

Mrs. Wilson thought for a moment and then said, "You know what? I have a spare key. You can borrow it until you find your own."

The Jenkins were relieved and grateful. "Thank you so much," said Mr. Jenkins. "We'll return it as soon as we find our key."

As they were about to enter their house, they noticed that their cat, Whiskers, was missing. They searched the house and the neighborhood, but there was no sign of him.

"We can't find Whiskers," said Mrs. Jenkins.

"Oh no, we have to find him," said Mr. Jenkins.

Just then, they saw their neighbor, Mr. Brown, walking his dog.

"Have you seen our cat, Whiskers?" asked Mrs. Jenkins.

"No, I haven't," replied Mr. Brown. "But I'll keep an eye out for him."

As they continued their search, they saw a little boy playing with a cat that looked just like Whiskers.

"Excuse me, is that your cat?" asked Mrs. Jenkins.

The boy nodded.

"That's our cat," said Mr. Jenkins.

The boy looked confused. "But he followed me home," he said.

The Jenkins realized that Whiskers must have followed the boy home by mistake.

"Thank you so much for finding him," said Mrs. Jenkins.

As they walked back to their house, they realized that they still had Mrs. Wilson's spare key. They knocked on her door, and she answered with a smile.

"We found our cat, but we still have your spare key," explained Mr. Jenkins.

"That's okay, keep it," said Mrs. Wilson. "You never know when you might need it again."

The Jenkins thanked Mrs. Wilson again and went inside their house, feeling grateful for their kind neighbors and relieved that they had found Whiskers.

As they sat down for a cup of tea, Mrs. Jenkins said, "It's amazing how everything worked out in the end."

"Yes, it is," agreed Mr. Jenkins. "Sometimes, all it takes is a little help from our friends."

The Colorful Music Box

In the heart of the bustling city, there stood an old antique store. Inside, there were many treasures waiting to be discovered. Among them, there was a music box that caught the eye of an old man named Mr. Thompson.

Mr. Thompson was an elderly man who enjoyed the simple things in life. He loved to reminisce about the past and often found himself lost in thought. The music box reminded him of his childhood, and he couldn't resist the urge to buy it.

As he walked out of the store, he noticed a young girl sitting on the sidewalk, playing a violin. She played with such passion and skill that it caught Mr. Thompson's attention. He stopped to listen, and the girl noticed him and smiled.

They struck up a conversation, and Mr. Thompson discovered that the girl's name was Lily, and she was an aspiring musician. She played on the streets to earn money to pay for her music lessons.

Moved by her talent and determination, Mr. Thompson offered to pay for her lessons. Lily was overjoyed and grateful for his kindness.

From that day on, they would meet regularly, and Mr. Thompson would listen to Lily play the violin. He loved how the music filled the air with color and brought back memories of his youth.

One day, Mr. Thompson brought the music box to their meeting. As he opened it, the most beautiful melody filled the air. The music box had a way of transporting him back in time, and he felt like a young boy again.

Lily was fascinated by the music box and asked if she could try playing her violin along with the melody. Mr. Thompson agreed, and as they played together, something magical happened. The music seemed to come alive, and the colors around them became brighter and more vivid.

As they finished playing, Mr. Thompson realized that the music box had the power to bring people together and create something beautiful. He decided to donate it to the local community center so that everyone could enjoy its magic.

In the end, Mr. Thompson and Lily continued to play music together, and their friendship grew stronger. The music box had brought them together and had given them a new sense of purpose and joy.

As Mr. Thompson walked home, he couldn't help but feel grateful for the memories that the music box had brought back. He realized that sometimes the simplest things in life can have the most profound impact.

The Old Barber's Secret

Mr. Potts was an old barber who had been cutting hair for over sixty years. He had seen it all, from the latest fashions to the worst hair disasters. But despite his long career, there was one secret that he had never told anyone.

One day, a young man came into Mr. Potts' barber shop. He had just started a new job and wanted to look his best. Mr. Potts listened to the young man's story and then got to work. As he cut the young man's hair, he began to tell him a story.

"Many years ago, when I was a young barber just starting out, I had a customer who asked me to shave his beard. I had never done it before, but I was eager to learn. So, I grabbed my razor and got to work. But then, something strange happened. The man's beard started to grow back right before my eyes. It was like magic."

The young man listened intently as Mr. Potts continued his story.

"The man looked at me and said, 'You have a gift, my boy. You can make hair grow.' And then he

Suddenly, Paddy's face lit up with recognition as he spotted an old friend in the crowd. They exchanged warm greetings and began to reminisce about old times. Tommy watched as his grandfather's eyes sparkled with delight and listened intently as they shared stories of their youth.

As they continued on their way, Tommy's attention was drawn to a group of elderly women, all dressed in green and chatting excitedly amongst themselves. They seemed to be having a wonderful time, and Tommy wondered what they were talking about.

"Excuse me, ma'am," he said to one of the women. "What are you all talking about?"

The woman smiled warmly and replied, "Oh, we're just reminiscing about our own St. Patrick's Day celebrations when we were young. It's wonderful to remember those happy times."

Tommy nodded, understandingly, and as they continued on their way, he found himself lost in thought. He wondered what memories he would have of this day when he grew older, and if he too would one day share those memories with his own grandchildren.

As they reached the end of the parade route, Tommy and Paddy sat down on a nearby bench to rest. Paddy leaned back, closing his eyes, and took a deep breath of the fresh spring air. Tommy watched as a smile spread across his grandfather's face, and he knew that he was thinking of all the happy times he had shared with his family and friends.

As the sun began to set, the parade ended with a spectacular display of fireworks. The colors and sounds filled the sky, and Tommy watched in awe as the explosions reflected in his grandfather's eyes.

"That was the best parade ever," he said, grinning from ear to ear.

Paddy chuckled softly and patted his grandson's hand. "Aye, lad, it was a grand day. But remember, the memories we make are what truly matter."

Tommy nodded thoughtfully, realizing that the sights and sounds of the day would fade, but the memories would last a lifetime.

As they made their way back home, Tommy felt a sense of contentment and joy, knowing that he had shared a special day with his grandfather and had created memories that would stay with him forever. The Colorful Parade had given him a glimpse of the past and a hope for the future, and he knew that he would always cherish this day.

The Musician's Legacy

In the bustling city of New Orleans, there was a small jazz club that had been around for generations. The club was called The Blue Note, and it was known for its lively atmosphere and the talented musicians who graced its stage.

One such musician was a man named Marcus, who had been playing at The Blue Note for over twenty years. Marcus was a master of the saxophone, and his smooth, sultry notes could bring tears to your eyes or make you want to get up and dance.

Over the years, Marcus had become a beloved fixture in the city, and people would come from all over to hear him play. He was a kind, gentle man who loved nothing more than sharing his music with others.

One evening, as Marcus was finishing up a set, a young woman approached him. She was holding a saxophone case and had a look of determination in her eyes.

"Excuse me, sir," she said. "I'm a musician, and I

was wondering if you could give me some advice."

Marcus smiled warmly at her and invited her to sit down. They talked for hours, discussing everything from music theory to the struggles of being a performer. As the night wore on, the woman realized that Marcus was not only a great musician but also a wise and generous mentor.

Over the next few years, the woman continued to visit Marcus at The Blue Note, and he watched as she grew and flourished as a musician. She eventually started her own band and began to play at venues all over the city.

One day, Marcus fell ill and was unable to play at The Blue Note for several weeks. The club was filled with people who came to see him, but they were disappointed to learn that he wouldn't be performing.

The young woman, now a successful musician in her own right, heard about Marcus's illness and knew that she had to do something to help. She organized a benefit concert at The Blue Note, and all the proceeds went toward Marcus's medical bills.

The concert was a huge success, and the club was filled with people who had come to show their support for Marcus. As the musicians played, Marcus sat in the audience, listening to the music with tears in his eyes.

After the concert, the young woman approached Marcus and handed him a check with the proceeds from the benefit. Marcus was overwhelmed with gratitude and knew that he had made a lasting impact on her life.

As the years went by, Marcus continued to play at The Blue Note, but he also became a mentor to many young musicians in the city. He passed down his knowledge and love of music to the next generation, ensuring that his legacy would live on.

Years later, when Marcus passed away, the city of New Orleans mourned the loss of a true legend. But his music and his spirit lived on, and young musicians would still come to The Blue Note, hoping to follow in his footsteps.

As the saxophone filled the air, people would close their eyes and listen to the smooth, sultry notes, and they knew that Marcus's legacy would never die.

The Missing Piece

Mrs. Thompson was an elderly woman who lived alone in a large house on the outskirts of town. She had been widowed for many years, and although she had friends and family who visited her from time to time, she often felt a sense of emptiness and longing.

One day, as she was walking in the woods behind her house, she stumbled upon a strange object. It was a large, flat stone with a hole in the center, and Mrs. Thompson couldn't help but feel drawn to it.

She picked up the stone and examined it closely, turning it over in her hands. She had never seen anything like it before, and she couldn't help but wonder what it was for.

As she made her way back to her house, the stone in her pocket, Mrs. Thompson felt a sense of excitement and curiosity. She spent the rest of the day researching online, trying to find out more about this mysterious object.

Over the next few weeks, Mrs. Thompson became obsessed with the stone. She carried it with her wherever she went, and she spent hours each day trying to fit different objects through the hole in the center.

At first, she tried small things like keys and coins, but they didn't fit. Then she tried larger objects like books and vases, but they didn't fit either.

But Mrs. Thompson was determined, and she refused to give up. She spent days and weeks trying to find the missing piece that would fit through the hole in the center of the stone.

As time went on, Mrs. Thompson's obsession with the stone began to worry her family and friends. They tried to convince her to put it down and move on with her life, but she couldn't let go.

Then, one day, something magical happened. As she was walking in the woods with the stone in her pocket, Mrs. Thompson stumbled upon a small piece of wood that was the perfect size to fit through the hole in the center of the stone.

She picked up the piece of wood and tried it in the hole, and it fit perfectly. Mrs. Thompson couldn't believe her luck, and she felt a sense of satisfaction and completeness that she had never felt before.

Over the next few days, Mrs. Thompson spent hours playing with the stone and the piece of wood, marveling at how they fit together so perfectly. She realized that the missing piece she had been searching for was not an object at all, but a feeling of completeness and belonging.

From that day on, Mrs. Thompson's life changed. She no longer felt the sense of emptiness and longing that had plagued her for so long. She had found the missing piece, and it was not something she could hold in her hand, but a sense of purpose and connection to the world around her.

As she grew older, Mrs. Thompson continued to carry the stone with her, but she no longer obsessed over finding the missing piece. She had learned that sometimes, the things we search for are not physical objects, but feelings that we carry within us.

The Golden Key

In the bustling city of New York, a young boy named Charlie lived with his grandfather. Charlie's grandfather was an old man who had lived a long and full life, but his memory was starting to fade. Charlie loved spending time with his grandfather and listening to his stories of the past, but he was worried that his grandfather would forget these precious memories.

One day, while exploring the city, Charlie stumbled upon a small antique shop. As he perused the shop's shelves, he came across a small, golden key. Intrigued, he asked the shopkeeper about it. The shopkeeper told him that the key was magical and had the power to unlock memories. Charlie was skeptical, but the shopkeeper insisted that the key was a valuable treasure.

Charlie decided to buy the key and brought it home to show his grandfather. At first, his grandfather was confused, but as soon as Charlie placed the key in his hand, something magical happened. Memories flooded back to him, and he began to tell Charlie stories of his past that he had forgotten.

The two of them spent hours unlocking memories with the golden key. They talked about old friends, long-lost loves, and the adventures they had experienced together. The more they used the key, the more vivid their memories became, and they felt closer than ever before.

As time passed, Charlie's grandfather's memory continued to fade, but they always had the golden key to help them remember. They passed the key down to Charlie's children and grandchildren, and it became a treasured family heirloom.

Years later, on Charlie's grandfather's 100th birthday, the whole family gathered together to celebrate. As they looked back on their memories, they all realized how important the golden key had been in keeping their family's history alive. They raised a glass to Charlie's grandfather and to the magic of the golden key, which had brought them all closer together.

In the end, Charlie realized that the true magic of the key wasn't in its ability to unlock memories, but in the memories themselves. He knew that as long as he and his family had each other and their memories, they would always be able to keep their past alive.

As the family said their goodbyes, Charlie's grandfather gave him one last piece of advice, "Hold on to your memories, Charlie, for they are the key to unlocking a life well-lived."

And so, the golden key became a symbol of the power of memories, and the importance of holding on to them. As the family left the party, Charlie slipped the key into his pocket, knowing that it would always be with him, a reminder of the love and memories that had brought them all together.

The Miracle of the Magnolia Tree

In a small town nestled among rolling hills, there was a majestic magnolia tree. Its branches reached high into the sky, and its fragrant flowers filled the air with their sweet aroma. The townspeople had always cherished the tree and believed that it held special powers.

One year, the town was hit by a severe drought. The crops were withering, and the people were afraid that they would run out of food. One day, an old man named Henry had an idea. He approached the town council and suggested that they pray to the magnolia tree for rain.

The council was skeptical, but Henry was insistent. He knew that the tree was a symbol of hope for the town and believed that it could perform a miracle. The townspeople agreed to follow Henry's lead and gathered around the magnolia tree to pray for rain.

Days passed, and there was no sign of rain. The people began to lose hope and wondered if Henry's idea was just a pipe dream. But then, something miraculous happened. A small cloud appeared on the horizon, and soon, rain began to fall from the sky.

The people rejoiced and credited the magnolia tree for the miracle. They believed that their prayers had been answered, and that the tree had somehow made it rain. From that day on, the magnolia tree became a symbol of faith and hope for the town.

Years went by, and the magnolia tree continued to thrive. It became a gathering place for the townspeople, who would sit under its shade and share stories of their lives. The tree became a witness to the joys and sorrows of the people, and they believed that it had a special connection to the divine.

One day, a young woman named Sarah moved to the town. She was new to the area and didn't know anyone. But when she saw the magnolia tree, she felt drawn to it. She would sit under its branches and talk to it as if it were a friend.

As time went on, Sarah became a part of the community. She made friends and found a job, but the magnolia tree remained her constant companion. She would share her dreams and hopes with the tree, and it seemed to listen.

One day, Sarah was walking home from work when she saw that the magnolia tree had been cut down. Its branches lay on the ground, and its trunk had been chopped into pieces. Sarah was devastated. She felt as if she had lost a dear friend.

The town council had decided that the tree was too old and posed a danger to the people. They had no choice but to cut it down. But Sarah knew that the tree had been much more than just a tree. It had been a symbol of faith and hope for the town, and a friend to all who had sought its shade.

As she stood there, looking at the remains of the magnolia tree, something miraculous happened. A small sapling sprouted from the ground where the tree had once stood. Its leaves were small and delicate, and its trunk was thin, but it was alive.

The townspeople saw the sapling and knew that it was a sign of hope. They believed that the magnolia tree had somehow passed on its powers to the sapling and that it would one day grow into a magnificent tree.

Sarah smiled and knew that the magnolia tree had given her a gift. It had taught her the power of faith and hope, and had shown her that even in the darkest of times, miracles could happen.

The Gift of Giving

Once upon a time, there was a kind-hearted man named Tom. Tom had always lived a simple life, content with what he had and never asking for more. He owned a small farm on the outskirts of town and spent his days tending to his crops and animals.

One day, as Tom was walking through the town square, he saw a group of children playing with a worn-out ball. He noticed how much joy the children were getting from this simple object, and it made him realize how fortunate he was to have all that he had. Tom decided that he wanted to give back to his community in a meaningful way.

Tom decided to donate his entire harvest to the local food bank, hoping to help those in need. His neighbors were surprised by his generosity, and some even tried to dissuade him, telling him that he needed to think of himself first. But Tom was determined to give what he could, and he knew that it was the right thing to do.

As the harvest season ended, Tom loaded up his wagon with his bounty and set off for the food bank. When he arrived, he was greeted with open arms by the volunteers who were overwhelmed by the amount of food he had brought. They thanked him profusely and assured him that his donation would make a real difference in the lives of those who needed it.

But the story doesn't end there. One evening, a few weeks after Tom's donation, there was a knock on his door. It was the local baker, who had been given some of Tom's crops by the food bank. The baker had baked a loaf of bread with Tom's flour and wanted to share it with him as a thank you.

Tom was touched by the baker's gesture and couldn't help but feel grateful for the kindness of others. He realized that by giving, he had received so much more in return. From that day on, Tom continued to give what he could to those in need, and he always received so much joy in return.

The Gift of Laughter

In the heart of the city, there was a small comedy club called "The Chuckle Factory". It was known for its hilarious stand-up comedy acts and had become a popular spot for locals and tourists alike. The owner of the club, Harry, was a jovial man with a heart of gold. He loved nothing more than to make people laugh and forget their troubles.

One night, a young man named Jack stumbled into the club. He was down on his luck and had nowhere else to go. Harry noticed Jack's gloomy demeanor and invited him to stay for the comedy show. Jack reluctantly agreed and took a seat in the back of the room.

As the night went on, Jack found himself laughing harder than he had in years. The comedians were so funny that he forgot all about his problems and felt like a weight had been lifted from his shoulders. When the show ended, Harry approached Jack and asked him what he thought.

"I haven't laughed like that in ages," Jack said. "Thank you for the gift of laughter."

Harry smiled and said, "You know, laughter is the best medicine. It can cure anything, even a broken heart."

From that night on, Jack visited The Chuckle Factory every week. He would sit in the front row and laugh until his sides hurt. Harry noticed the change in Jack's demeanor and was thrilled that he could make such a difference in someone's life.

One day, Harry received a letter from Jack. It was an invitation to his wedding. Jack had met the love of his life, and he credited Harry and The Chuckle Factory with bringing laughter and happiness back into his life.

Harry attended the wedding and was honored to be a part of Jack's special day. As he watched Jack and his bride exchange vows, he knew that he had found his true calling in life. He wanted to bring joy and laughter to as many people as possible.

Years passed, and Harry continued to run The Chuckle Factory. He became a beloved figure in the city, and people would come from far and wide to see the comedy acts. Harry knew that he had found his purpose in life, and he was grateful for the gift of laughter that he had been able to share with so many.

One day, as Harry was closing up the club, he noticed a young man sitting on the steps outside. He looked lost and dejected. Harry approached him and asked him what was wrong.

"I just lost my job," the young man said. "I don't know what to do."

Harry smiled and said, "Well, you're in luck. You're at The Chuckle Factory, the home of laughter. Let me buy you a ticket to tonight's show. I promise it'll make you forget all about your troubles."

The young man hesitated for a moment but then nodded his head. As he walked into the club, he heard the sound of laughter and knew that he had found a place where he belonged. And Harry knew that he had once again given someone the gift of laughter.

The Lucky Penny

Maggie was a hard-working woman who lived in a small town in the countryside. She owned a modest bakery, which she had inherited from her parents. She loved baking, and she worked tirelessly to create delicious treats for her customers. Despite her long hours and hard work, she struggled to make ends meet, and money was always tight.

One day, while taking a walk in the town square, Maggie spotted a shiny penny on the ground. She picked it up and looked at it closely. It was a 1943 penny, a rare coin that was worth a lot of money. Maggie couldn't believe her luck. She had always been a bit superstitious, and finding a lucky penny was a sign that good things were on the horizon.

Maggie decided to keep the penny with her at all times, hoping that it would bring her good fortune. And to her surprise, things did start to look up. Her business began to grow, and her loyal customers continued to spread the word about her delicious treats.

One day, a man named Jack came into her bakery. He was new to town and was looking for a job. Maggie was in need of some help around the bakery, and Jack seemed like the perfect fit. She hired him on the spot, and they quickly became good friends.

As they worked together in the bakery, Jack and Maggie would often chat about their lives and their dreams. Jack was an artist, and he had always dreamed of painting murals in big cities like New York and Paris. Maggie listened with fascination, admiring Jack's creativity and his passion for art.

One day, Jack showed Maggie some of his paintings, and she was blown away by their beauty. They were unlike anything she had ever seen before, full of color and life. Maggie was convinced that Jack's paintings could make a real impact in the art world, and she encouraged him to pursue his dream of painting murals.

At first, Jack was hesitant. He didn't have the money or the connections to make it in the art world. But Maggie reminded him of the lucky penny and how it had brought her good fortune. She urged him to take a chance and to believe in himself.

With Maggie's encouragement, Jack applied for a grant to fund his mural project. To his amazement, he was awarded the grant, and he set off for New York to paint his first mural. Maggie was thrilled for him and couldn't wait to see his masterpiece.

Months went by, and Maggie continued to run her bakery. She missed Jack's company and his artistic flair, but she knew that he was living his dream. One day, she received a package in the mail from Jack. Inside was a beautiful painting of the two of them standing in front of the bakery. The painting was full of color and life, just like Jack's murals.

Maggie was overwhelmed with emotion. She couldn't believe that Jack had painted such a beautiful tribute to their friendship. And then she noticed something in the corner of the painting. It was a shiny penny, the same lucky penny that had brought her good fortune. She smiled to herself, feeling grateful for the small things in life that could bring so much joy.

From that day on, Maggie continued to run her bakery with joy and passion, knowing that good things were always on the horizon.

The Sweetness of Generosity

It was a sweltering summer day when young Joey decided to open a lemonade stand in front of his grandfather's house. With a pitcher of fresh lemonade and a handful of cups, he set up shop under the shade of a big oak tree.

As he waited for customers to come, he watched the world go by. He saw the mailman making his rounds, the neighbors walking their dogs, and children playing in the street. The sound of laughter and chatter filled the air, and Joey felt happy to be a part of it all.

Suddenly, an old man hobbled up to the stand. He was bent over with age, and his face was lined with wrinkles. Joey greeted him with a smile, and the man looked at him with a twinkle in his eye.

"Sonny, do you have any iced tea?" the old man asked.

Joey shook his head. "Sorry, sir. All I have is lemonade."

The old man sighed. "I used to love iced tea

when I was your age. But now, my taste buds don't work so well anymore. I can't taste the sweetness."

Joey felt a pang of sadness in his heart. He wanted to make the old man happy. So, he grabbed a bottle of honey from his backpack and added a spoonful to the lemonade.

"Here, try this," Joey said, handing the old man a cup.

The old man took a sip, and a smile spread across his face. "My goodness, this is the best lemonade I've ever tasted!"

Joey felt a sense of pride and accomplishment. He had made someone happy with his lemonade. From that moment on, he knew that he wanted to make people happy for the rest of his life.

As the day wore on, Joey's lemonade stand became the talk of the town. People came from far and wide just to taste his delicious lemonade. Even the mayor stopped by to have a cup.

But as the sun began to set, Joey realized that he had run out of lemons. He was about to close up shop when the old man returned.

"Sonny, I have a surprise for you," the old man said, handing Joey a small bag.

Joey opened the bag and gasped. It was full of lemons!

"Where did you get these?" Joey asked in amazement.

"I used to have a lemon tree in my yard," the old man replied. "But I'm too old to take care of it now. I figured you could put them to better use."

Joey felt a surge of gratitude in his heart. He knew that this was a sign of the goodness of humanity. He decided to donate a portion of his earnings to help the elderly man.

From that day on, Joey's lemonade stand became a staple of the community. He always had a smile on his face and a kind word for everyone who came by. And every time he squeezed a lemon, he thought of the old man who had taught him the true meaning of generosity and kindness.

As he grew older, Joey became a successful businessman. But he never forgot his humble beginnings as a lemonade stand owner. He always remembered the lessons he had learned from the old man, and he passed them on to his own children and grandchildren.

Years later, when Joey was an old man himself, he sat under the same oak tree where he had once set up his lemonade stand. The sound of laughter and chatter filled the air, just like it had on that hot summer day. And as he closed his eyes and took a deep breath, he could almost taste the sweetness of the lemonade, and feel the warmth of the sun on his skin.

The Sweetest Things in Life

It was a warm summer day, and Mr. Jameson, a retired candy maker, was taking a leisurely walk through the streets of his old neighborhood. The sights and sounds of the bustling city filled him with a sense of nostalgia, and he couldn't help but feel a twinge of sadness at the thought of all the memories he had left behind. As he walked past the old candy shop where he had spent so many happy years, he couldn't help but smile at the thought of all the sweet memories it held.

As he continued his walk, he found himself in front of a small park. He noticed a young boy sitting on a bench, staring intently at a butterfly perched on his finger. Mr. Jameson approached the boy and asked him if he liked candy. The boy nodded eagerly, and Mr. Jameson reached into his pocket and pulled out a small bag of his famous peppermint drops. The boy's eyes widened in delight as he took a handful and popped one into his mouth. The sweet, refreshing taste filled his mouth, and he let out a happy sigh.

Mr. Jameson sat down next to the boy, and they struck up a conversation. The boy told him about his dreams of becoming a scientist, and Mr. Jameson told him about his own experiences as a candy maker. They talked for hours, lost in the joy of each other's company.

As the sun began to set, Mr. Jameson stood up to leave. The boy thanked him for the candy and the conversation, and Mr. Jameson thanked him for reminding him of the sweetest things in life. As he walked away, he couldn't help but feel a sense of happiness and contentment. He had been reminded of the joy of sharing, of connecting with others, and of the simple pleasures that make life worth living.

That night, as he sat in his favorite armchair, Mr. Jameson thought back on his long and fulfilling life. He had experienced many highs and lows, but he realized that the sweetest moments had always been the ones spent in the company of others, sharing laughter and conversation over a bag of his famous peppermint drops. As he drifted off to sleep, a smile on his face, he knew that he had lived a life filled with love and joy.

The Gift of the Magi

Della and Jim were a young couple deeply in love, but struggling to make ends meet. As Christmas approached, Della became determined to find the perfect gift for Jim. She longed to give him something truly special, but with only a few dollars to her name, she knew it would be a challenge.

As she walked the streets of New York City, she passed a luxurious hair salon and was struck with an idea. She would sell her long, beautiful hair to a wig maker, and use the money to buy Jim a watch chain for his beloved pocket watch. Della's heart raced with excitement as she imagined the look of delight on Jim's face when he opened the gift.

Meanwhile, Jim was struggling to come up with the perfect gift for Della. He had a treasured gold watch that had been passed down through his family for generations, but it was useless without a chain. He knew that a chain would be the perfect gift for Della, but he had no money to buy one.

On Christmas Eve, Della and Jim exchanged gifts. As Della revealed her short, cropped hair to Jim, he was taken aback. He couldn't help but feel a pang of guilt that he had not been able to give her the beautiful gifts she deserved.

But as he pulled out the small, simple chain he had bought for her, Della's eyes lit up with joy. She embraced Jim tightly, tears streaming down her face. Jim couldn't help but feel a sense of wonder and amazement at the sacrifices they had both made for each other.

As they sat together in the quiet of their small apartment, they realized that the true gift of Christmas was not in the material possessions they had given each other, but in the love they shared. They had given each other the greatest gift of all - the gift of selfless love and sacrifice.

Memories on the Corner

In the heart of New York City, on a bustling street, lived a young couple named Jack and Mary. They had just moved to the city from a small town, and they were still adjusting to the fast-paced life of the city.

One day, while walking through the park, they stumbled upon an old man sitting on a bench, staring at a tree. The man looked up and smiled at them, and they noticed his kind eyes and gentle demeanor. They struck up a conversation with the man, and he told them about his life and his love for the park.

The old man, whose name was George, soon became a regular fixture in Jack and Mary's life. They would often bring him sandwiches and coffee, and they would sit and chat with him for hours on end.

One day, George took them to a little ice cream shop that he loved. The shop was old-fashioned, with a long counter and stools, and the walls were lined with pictures of the city in the 1920s. The shop had an assortment of flavors, from classic vanilla to exotic combinations like lavender and honey.

As they sat at the counter, enjoying their ice cream, George told them stories of his youth and how he would come to this shop with his friends. He talked about the sights, sounds, and smells of the city in the old days, and he recounted the adventures he had with his friends.

Jack and Mary listened intently, their imaginations sparked by George's vivid descriptions. They could almost smell the hot dogs and roasted peanuts from the street vendors, and they could hear the sounds of the streetcars and the chatter of people.

As they were leaving the shop, George handed them a small paper bag. "For later," he said with a wink. When they got home, they opened the bag to find a handful of old-fashioned candies that George had bought for them.

Jack and Mary were touched by the gesture, and they realized how much George had become a part of their lives. They went back to the ice cream shop the next day, and the next, and they brought George with them every time.

As the days went by, Jack and Mary noticed that

George seemed to be getting younger. His eyes sparkled with mischief, and he had a spring in his step that hadn't been there before. They also noticed that he seemed to be forgetting things, like the name of the park or the flavor of his ice cream.

One day, as they were walking through the park, George suddenly stopped and looked around. "Where am I?" he asked, his eyes wide with confusion. Jack and Mary realized with a pang that George had Alzheimer's disease.

They continued to visit George, bringing him ice cream and candies, and listening to his stories. Even as his memory faded, he still had a twinkle in his eye and a mischievous grin.

One day, as they were leaving the ice cream shop, George handed them a small paper bag. "For later," he said with a wink. When they got home, they opened the bag to find a note from George. It read:

"Dear Jack and Mary,
Thank you for the sweetest surprise of my life. Your kindness and friendship have kept my memories alive, and I will cherish them always.
With love,
George"

Jack and Mary smiled through their tears, grateful for the time they had spent with George and the memories they had created together. They knew that they would never forget the sweet old man who had become such an important part of their lives.

The Musician's Gift

It was a typical Saturday morning in the small town of Millville. The sun was shining, and the birds were singing, as people went about their business. Among them was a young girl named Lily, who loved nothing more than to play her violin.

Lily had been playing the violin since she was six years old. Her parents had recognized her talent early on and had encouraged her to pursue music. Lily had taken to the violin like a fish to water, and soon, she was playing in recitals and competitions.

One day, as Lily was practicing in the park, an old man approached her. He was carrying a battered guitar, and his clothes were threadbare. Lily didn't think much of it at first, but as the man started to play, she realized that he was a talented musician.

Lily listened intently as the man played his guitar, and she noticed the way his fingers danced over the strings. She saw the joy on his face as he played, and she realized that music was not just something she loved to do, it was something that brought happiness to others.

From that day on, Lily started playing in the park with the old man. They played together every Saturday morning, and people would gather around to listen. They played old folk songs and classical pieces, and Lily would often improvise on her violin while the old man strummed his guitar.

As they played, Lily noticed that the old man's clothes were getting shabbier, and his guitar was starting to fall apart. She knew that he couldn't afford to buy a new guitar, and she wanted to do something to help.

Lily decided to organize a benefit concert for the old man. She spread the word around town and enlisted the help of her fellow musicians. They spent weeks practicing, and soon, they had put together an amazing concert.

The day of the concert arrived, and Lily was nervous but excited. The concert was held in the town square, and people came from all over to listen. The musicians played their hearts out, and the old man was the star of the show.

At the end of the concert, Lily presented the old man with a brand new guitar. Tears streamed down his face as he thanked Lily and the other musicians. He hugged Lily and told her that she had given him the gift of music.

From that day on, the old man played his guitar with renewed passion, and Lily continued to play her violin with joy in her heart. They continued to play together in the park, and people would often stop to listen and marvel at the magic of their music.

Years went by, and Lily grew up to become a professional musician. She played in orchestras and traveled all over the world, but she never forgot the old man and the gift of music he had given her.

Whenever she returned to Millville, Lily would visit the old man in the park, and they would play together once again. They had both grown older, but their love of music had never faded.

As Lily played her violin and the old man strummed his guitar, the people in the park would stop and listen, their faces filled with wonder and joy. And Lily knew that, just like the old man had given her the gift of music, she was now passing it on to a new generation of listeners.

The Time Traveler

Once upon a time, in a small town tucked away in the countryside, there lived a young man named Peter. Peter was not like most young men his age. He had a special gift that no one else had - the ability to time travel. One moment he would be in the present day, and the next he would be transported back to a different time and place altogether.

One day, Peter woke up feeling particularly nostalgic. He decided to use his gift to travel back to his childhood home, where he had spent many happy years with his family. As he closed his eyes and concentrated on the place he wanted to go, he felt a strange sensation wash over him, and he suddenly found himself standing outside his old house.

Peter walked around the familiar streets, taking in the sights and sounds of his childhood. He visited his old school, the park where he used to play with his friends, and even the corner store where he used to buy his favorite candy. Everything was just as he remembered it - the bright colors, the smells of freshly cut grass and baked goods, the sound of children's laughter echoing through the streets.

As Peter walked, he encountered many old friends and acquaintances, all of whom were now much older. They marveled at how young and energetic Peter seemed, and he enjoyed reminiscing with them about old times. They shared stories of their past adventures, and Peter found himself laughing at the silly things they used to do.

As the day wore on, Peter felt a sense of contentment wash over him. He realized that even though he had traveled back in time, he was still the same person he had always been. The memories and experiences he had accumulated over the years had shaped him into the person he was today, and he was grateful for every moment of it.

As the sun began to set and the sky turned a deep shade of orange, Peter knew it was time to return to the present day. He closed his eyes and concentrated once more, and when he opened them again, he was back in his own time. He smiled to himself, feeling a sense of satisfaction and happiness wash over him.

From that day forward, Peter made it a point to use his time-traveling gift to visit different places and times throughout his life. Each time he traveled, he gained a new appreciation for the memories and experiences that had shaped him into the person he was today. And even though he was now an old man, his memories kept him young at heart and filled with a sense of wonder and joy.

The Dancing Queen

In a small retirement home on the outskirts of town, there lived a woman named Martha. Martha had lived a long and fulfilling life, but now that she was in her golden years, she often found herself feeling bored and lonely. She longed for the days when she could dance and move freely, but her old bones wouldn't allow her to do so anymore.

One day, the retirement home decided to host a dance party for its residents, and Martha couldn't contain her excitement. She put on her best dress and makeup, and as soon as the music started playing, she was on the dance floor, moving and grooving to the beat.

At first, the other residents looked on in amusement as Martha twirled and dipped, but soon enough, they too found themselves joining in. The room was filled with laughter and joy as the residents danced and sang along to their favorite tunes.

Martha felt alive again, like she was back in her youth. She closed her eyes and let the music wash over her, feeling grateful for this moment of pure happiness.

As the night went on, Martha danced with everyone - the other residents, the staff, even the volunteers. She felt like a queen, ruling over her kingdom of dancers.

Finally, as the night drew to a close and the music slowed down, Martha found herself swaying in the arms of a handsome gentleman. She looked up at him and smiled, feeling a flutter in her heart that she hadn't felt in years.

As the dance ended, the gentleman leaned in and whispered in her ear, "You dance like a queen."

Martha felt a warm blush spread across her cheeks as she thanked him. She knew that even though she was old and her body wasn't what it used to be, she still had the spirit of a dancer inside her.

From that day forward, Martha made it a point to dance every chance she got. Whether it was at the weekly dance parties at the retirement home or just in her own room, she never let her age stop her from doing what she loved.

And whenever she danced, she felt like a queen,

ruling over her own kingdom of joy and happiness.

The Art of Giving

Mrs. Margaret Johnson had lived in the same house on Elm Street for over fifty years. She had raised her family there, and it was the place where she had made countless memories. But as she grew older, the house had become too big for her, and she knew it was time to downsize.

Margaret was a talented painter, and her house was filled with her artwork. She knew that she couldn't take all her paintings with her when she moved, so she decided to have an art sale. She would sell her paintings and donate the money to charity.

Margaret spent weeks preparing for the sale. She cleaned and organized her paintings, and she made signs to put up around town. On the day of the sale, Margaret's yard was filled with people browsing through her paintings.

Among the crowd was a young girl named Sophie. Sophie loved art, and she had begged her parents to take her to the sale. Sophie had saved up her allowance for weeks, and she was hoping to find a painting that she could afford.

Sophie was walking through the yard, looking at the paintings, when she saw a painting that caught her eye. It was a beautiful landscape painting of a meadow filled with wildflowers. Sophie knew that she had to have it.

But when Sophie asked the price, Margaret told her that it was out of her budget. Sophie was disappointed, but she understood. She walked away, hoping that she might find something else that she liked.

As Sophie was leaving, Margaret stopped her. "Wait a minute," she said. "I have an idea." Margaret took Sophie's hand and led her into the house.

In the living room, Margaret showed Sophie a pile of blank canvases. "I have always believed that art should be accessible to everyone," Margaret said. "So, I am going to teach you how to paint."

Sophie was overjoyed. Margaret spent the whole afternoon teaching her how to mix colors and how to hold the brush. They worked together on a painting of the meadow, and Sophie was amazed at how quickly she was learning.

As the sun was setting, Margaret presented Sophie with the painting they had worked on together. "This is my gift to you," she said. "It's not the original, but it's just as beautiful."

Sophie was thrilled. She hugged Margaret and promised to keep painting. Margaret watched as Sophie left, feeling grateful that she had been able to share her love of art with someone else.

Months went by, and Margaret moved into a smaller house. Her paintings were sold, and the money was donated to charity. But Margaret didn't feel sad. She had gained something much more valuable than money. She had gained the joy of giving.

And Sophie continued to paint. She would often think of Margaret and the gift she had given her. Sophie's paintings were filled with the colors and beauty that she had learned from Margaret. And she knew that, just like Margaret had given her the gift of art, she was now passing it on to others.

The Last Dance

The sun was setting over the quiet town, casting a warm golden light on the small park. In the center of the park, a band was playing lively music, and couples were dancing on the makeshift dance floor. Among them, an elderly man stood out, dressed in a sharp suit and a fedora hat. His name was Jack, and he was the best dancer in town.

As Jack twirled his partner around the dance floor, he felt a sense of joy and nostalgia wash over him. The music, the laughter, the smell of freshly cut grass - they all reminded him of his youth, of a time when he was carefree and full of life.

Suddenly, a familiar face appeared in the crowd. It was his old flame, Mary, looking as beautiful as ever. Jack's heart skipped a beat as he approached her, his hand outstretched.

"May I have this dance?" he asked, his voice filled with emotion.

Mary smiled and took his hand, and they began to move to the rhythm of the music. As they danced, they reminisced about old times, of the dances they had shared, the moments they had spent together.

For a brief moment, they were young again, and nothing else mattered. The world around them disappeared, and they were lost in their own memories.

As the song came to an end, Jack and Mary shared a tender embrace. It was a moment they would never forget, a moment of pure happiness and contentment.

As Jack walked away from the dance floor, he couldn't help but feel grateful for the experience. He realized that no matter how old he was, there was still joy and love to be found in life. And he knew that he would cherish this memory for the rest of his days.

As he left the park, he looked back at the dance floor, where couples were still moving to the music. He smiled to himself, knowing that he had lived a good life, filled with love and laughter.

And as he walked into the sunset, he felt a sense of peace and fulfillment, knowing that he had one last dance to remember.

The Magnificent Adventure of Mrs. Abigail

Mrs. Abigail was an elderly lady who lived in a small cottage near a beautiful meadow. She had a passion for adventure, and her days were filled with memories of the travels she had once enjoyed. One bright morning, she woke up with a sparkle in her eyes and decided it was time to embark on a new adventure.

She packed a small bag and headed to the train station. As she sat on the train, she watched the beautiful countryside pass by, feeling a sense of nostalgia and wonder. When the train stopped at a small station, Mrs. Abigail stepped out and began to explore the town.

She walked through the streets, admiring the colorful houses and the vibrant flowers that adorned them. She listened to the sweet melody of the birds singing and the sound of the children playing. She smelled the delicious aroma of fresh bread coming from a nearby bakery and the sweet fragrance of the blooming flowers. All these sensations filled her with joy, and she felt alive once again.

As she wandered around, she met a group of friendly locals who welcomed her with open arms. They showed her around the town, taking her to the most beautiful places and telling her stories about the history and culture of their town.

Mrs. Abigail felt a sense of belonging as she listened to their stories and shared her own. She laughed and talked with them, enjoying the warmth of their company. She realized that even though she was far from home, she had found a new family in this beautiful town.

As the day drew to a close, Mrs. Abigail sat on a bench overlooking a picturesque view of the town. She felt a sense of peace and contentment as she watched the sun set behind the mountains. She thought about her journey and realized that even though it was a short one, it had been a magnificent adventure.

As she made her way back to her cottage, Mrs. Abigail felt a renewed sense of purpose. She knew that there were still many adventures to be had, and she was determined to live life to the fullest.

She smiled to herself, feeling grateful for the wonderful day she had spent in the company of new friends. She knew that she had created memories that would last a lifetime and that she would cherish them forever.

The Surprise Visitor

Mrs. Miriam sat on her front porch, enjoying the warm sunshine and the peacefulness of her garden. As she sipped her tea, she noticed a young woman walking down the street, looking lost and confused.

Mrs. Miriam immediately got up and walked over to the woman. "Excuse me, dear, do you need any help?" she asked kindly.

The young woman looked up at her, tears in her eyes. "Yes, please," she said, her voice trembling. "I'm trying to find my grandmother's house, but I seem to have gotten lost."

Mrs. Miriam smiled and took the woman's hand. "Don't worry, dear, I know this town like the back of my hand. Let me help you find your way."

Together, they walked down the street, Mrs. Miriam pointing out the sights and sounds of the town. She talked about the history of the town and the different neighborhoods, and the young woman listened intently, amazed by the wealth of knowledge that Mrs. Miriam possessed.

As they turned a corner, the young woman suddenly stopped in her tracks. "That's it!" she exclaimed, pointing to a small cottage at the end of the street. "That's my grandmother's house!"

Mrs. Miriam smiled, happy to have been able to help. "I'm glad we found it," she said. "Do you want me to walk you to the door?"

The young woman shook her head. "No, that's okay," she said. "Thank you so much for your help. You're such a kind lady."

Mrs. Miriam smiled and watched as the young woman walked towards the cottage. As she turned to leave, she heard a voice calling out to her.

"Miriam! Miriam, is that you?"

She turned around and saw a familiar face, her old friend Martha, standing on the doorstep of the cottage.

Mrs. Miriam's eyes widened in surprise. "Martha, is that really you?" she asked, feeling a rush of emotions.

Martha walked over to her, a big smile on her face. "Yes, it's me! I was visiting my granddaughter for the weekend, and I never expected to see you here!"

The two women hugged, tears of joy streaming down their faces. They sat down on the porch and caught up on all that had happened in their lives since they had last met.

As they talked, Mrs. Miriam realized that sometimes, unexpected surprises can bring the greatest joy. She felt grateful for the chance encounter with the young woman, which had led to her reunion with her dear friend Martha.

As the sun began to set, Mrs. Miriam hugged Martha once more and said goodbye. She walked back to her porch, feeling a sense of contentment and happiness that she had not felt in a long time.

She knew that life was full of surprises, both big and small, and she was grateful for every one of them. She smiled to herself, feeling grateful for the joy that this unexpected encounter had brought into her life.

The Mysterious Package

Mrs. Gertrude had just turned 85, and she was feeling down. Her children and grandchildren lived far away, and she had been feeling lonely lately. But on this particular day, she received a mysterious package in the mail.

As she opened the package, she saw that it was a beautifully wrapped gift, with a note attached to it. The note read: "To Gertrude, from a secret admirer. Happy birthday!"

Mrs. Gertrude couldn't believe it. She had never had a secret admirer before, and she was thrilled at the thought. She quickly unwrapped the gift and saw that it was a beautiful, antique necklace.

She put the necklace on, admiring how it looked against her skin. She felt a rush of excitement and wondered who her secret admirer could be. She spent the rest of the day trying to figure it out, but she couldn't come up with any ideas.

The next day, she received another package in the mail, again from her secret admirer. This time, it was a box of her favorite chocolates.

Mrs. Gertrude smiled to herself, feeling happy and grateful for this mysterious person who was making her feel loved and appreciated. She spent the day enjoying the chocolates and feeling grateful for the joy that this unexpected surprise had brought into her life.

Over the next few days, Mrs. Gertrude received more packages from her secret admirer. There were flowers, books, and even a beautiful scarf. Each gift brought a smile to her face and made her feel loved and appreciated.

Finally, on the seventh day, Mrs. Gertrude received a package with a note attached to it. The note read: "To Gertrude, from your children and grandchildren. Happy birthday! We love you!"

Mrs. Gertrude couldn't believe it. Her children and grandchildren had planned this whole surprise for her, sending her gifts every day to make her feel loved and appreciated on her special day. She felt overwhelmed with gratitude and happiness, and tears streamed down her face.

As she sat in her living room, surrounded by the gifts from her family and her secret admirer, she realized that sometimes, the most wonderful surprises can come from the people we love the most.

She felt grateful for her family and for the love and joy that they brought into her life. And she knew that, no matter how far away they were, they would always be there for her when she needed them.

The Unexpected Visitor

Mr. Thompson was 92 years old, and he had lived alone for many years. He was content with his quiet life, but he often felt lonely and wished he had someone to talk to.

One day, while sitting in his favorite chair and reading a book, he heard a knock at the door. He wasn't expecting any visitors, but he got up and made his way to the door.

As he opened it, he saw a young woman standing on his doorstep. She had a kind smile on her face, and she introduced herself as Emily.

"Hello, Mr. Thompson," she said. "I'm from the local high school, and I'm here as part of a volunteer program. We're visiting seniors in the community, and I wanted to stop by and say hello."

Mr. Thompson was surprised but pleased to see a young person taking an interest in his well-being. He invited Emily inside, and they sat down in the living room.

As they talked, Mr. Thompson found himself opening up to Emily in a way that he hadn't with anyone in years. She listened to his stories and shared her own, and they found that they had a lot in common despite their age difference.

Over the next few weeks, Emily visited Mr. Thompson regularly. They would talk about everything from books to politics to their favorite memories. Mr. Thompson looked forward to her visits and felt a renewed sense of purpose and connection in his life.

Eventually, the volunteer program came to an end, and Emily had to say goodbye to Mr. Thompson. He was sad to see her go, but he was grateful for the time they had spent together.

As he sat in his living room, thinking about the unexpected visitor who had brought so much joy into his life, Mr. Thompson realized that sometimes, the most wonderful surprises come from the people we least expect.

He felt grateful for Emily and for the new perspective that she had given him on life. And he knew that, even though they may not see each other again, she had left a lasting impact on his heart.

The Gift of Music

Mrs. Jenkins was 87 years old, and she had always loved music. She had played the piano since she was a little girl and had never lost her passion for it.

However, in recent years, her hands had started to shake, and she found it difficult to play as well as she used to. She felt frustrated and sad that she couldn't enjoy her favorite hobby as much as she used to.

One day, while sitting in her living room, she heard a knock at the door. She opened it to find a group of young musicians standing outside.

"Hello, Mrs. Jenkins," one of them said. "We're from the local music school, and we heard that you used to play the piano. We were wondering if we could play some music for you."

Mrs. Jenkins was surprised but delighted at the offer. She invited them inside, and they set up their instruments in her living room.

As they started to play, Mrs. Jenkins felt a rush of emotion. The music was beautiful, and it brought back memories of when she used to play herself. She closed her eyes and let the music wash over her, feeling grateful for the gift of music that these young people had brought into her life.

After they finished playing, the musicians thanked Mrs. Jenkins and prepared to leave. But before they left, one of them handed her a small package.

"We have a gift for you," she said. "It's a recording of us playing some of our favorite pieces. We hope it brings you as much joy as you've brought us."

Mrs. Jenkins thanked them and watched as they left her home. She couldn't wait to listen to the recording and relive the wonderful music that they had played for her.

As she sat in her living room, holding the recording in her hand, Mrs. Jenkins realized that sometimes, the most wonderful gifts can come from unexpected places. She felt grateful for the young musicians who had brought music back into her life and for the joy that it had brought her.

And she knew that, no matter how old she got, music would always be a part of her soul.

The Colors of Memory

It was a warm summer evening when old Mr. Jenkins decided to take a stroll through the town. He had been feeling a little down lately, and he thought a change of scenery might help lift his spirits. As he walked, he took in the sights and sounds of the town he had called home for so many years. The smell of freshly baked bread from the bakery on the corner filled his nostrils, and the sound of children laughing and playing in the park brought a smile to his face.

As he made his way down Main Street, he heard a familiar voice calling his name. It was Mrs. Thompson, his neighbor from down the street. She had a big grin on her face and waved excitedly as she approached him.

"Mr. Jenkins! What a lovely evening for a walk. Would you like some company?"

He nodded and they continued down the street together, chatting and laughing like old friends. As they walked, Mrs. Thompson pointed out various landmarks and buildings that had been there for as long as they could remember.

"Do you remember when the old cinema was still open? We used to go there every Saturday night."

Mr. Jenkins smiled wistfully. "Yes, and the smell of the popcorn and the sound of the projector starting up. It was always a special treat."

As they walked, memories flooded back to him. The bright colors of the marquee, the crunch of the popcorn, the feeling of excitement as the lights dimmed and the movie began. He felt alive again, and grateful for this unexpected walk down memory lane.

They continued their stroll, eventually making their way to the town square where a small band was playing music. Couples were dancing under the twinkling lights, and the air was filled with the sounds of laughter and joy.

Mrs. Thompson turned to Mr. Jenkins, a mischievous twinkle in her eye. "Shall we dance?"

Without hesitation, Mr. Jenkins took her hand and they joined the throng of people swaying to the music. It had been years since he had danced, but he found that his body remembered the steps as if it had been yesterday. He felt invigorated and alive, as if a weight had been lifted from his shoulders.

As the night wore on, the music slowed and the crowd began to disperse. Mr. Jenkins and Mrs. Thompson made their way back home, tired but happy.

As he lay in bed that night, Mr. Jenkins thought about the evening he had just experienced. He realized that despite his age, he still had so much life left in him. He was grateful for the memories that had been stirred up, and for the joy that had been rekindled.

The colors of memory, he thought to himself. They never fade, and they always bring a smile to my face.

And with that, he closed his eyes and drifted off to sleep, content in the knowledge that he had lived a full and vibrant life.

The Unexpected Encounter

It was a quiet afternoon at the park when a young girl named Lily stumbled upon an old man sitting on a bench, staring out into the distance. He seemed lost in thought, and Lily couldn't help but be curious.

"Hello, sir," she said timidly, approaching the bench. "Do you mind if I sit here?"

The old man looked up, startled by her presence. He regarded her for a moment before nodding his head, gesturing for her to sit down.

They sat in silence for a while, the only sound the rustling of leaves in the wind. Lily fidgeted nervously, unsure of what to say to the stranger next to her.

Finally, the old man spoke. "Do you know what I'm thinking about, young lady?"

Lily shook her head.

"I'm thinking about all the things I wish I had done differently in my life. All the missed opportunities, the chances I didn't take. It's a heavy burden to carry."

Lily looked at him with sadness in her eyes. "I'm sorry, sir. That sounds really tough."

The old man smiled at her. "But you know what? Sitting here, talking to you, I feel like maybe it's not too late. Maybe there are still adventures to be had, new people to meet. Maybe I still have some living left to do."

Lily's face lit up with excitement. "That's right! You can still do anything you want, no matter how old you are."

The old man chuckled. "You're right, young lady. And maybe I'll start by trying something new. Like what, you ask? I don't know yet, but I have a feeling that something exciting is just around the corner."

As they sat there, watching the world go by, Lily felt a connection with the old man. He had lived a full life, and yet he still had so much to look forward to. She felt grateful for the unexpected encounter, and for the reminder that it's never too late to start something new.

As they parted ways, the old man turned to her and said, "Thank you, Lily. You may not realize it, but you've given me a new lease on life. I'll never forget this conversation."

Lily smiled at him, feeling a sense of satisfaction that she had helped someone else. As she walked away, she knew that the memory of this encounter would stay with her for a long time to come.

The Lasting Friendship

Mr. Thomas had lived in the same house on Maple Street for over fifty years. He knew everyone in the neighborhood, and everyone knew him. He was a friendly man, always willing to lend a hand or listen to someone's problems.

One day, a new family moved in next door. Mr. Thomas watched as they unloaded their furniture and boxes, curious about his new neighbors. He decided to welcome them to the neighborhood, so he put on his coat and walked next door.

"Hello there!" he called out, waving a hand.

The family turned to look at him, and a woman stepped forward to greet him. "Hi! I'm Sarah. We just moved in. Nice to meet you."

Mr. Thomas smiled at her. "Welcome to the neighborhood. My name is Thomas, but everyone calls me Mr. Thomas."

Over the next few weeks, Mr. Thomas and Sarah became good friends. They would sit on the porch and chat over cups of tea, sharing stories about their lives. Mr. Thomas was impressed by Sarah's intelligence and her kind heart, and he felt lucky to have her as a neighbor.

One day, Sarah came over to his house with a small box in her hand. "I wanted to give you something," she said, handing him the box.

Mr. Thomas opened it to find a beautiful handmade scarf inside. "Sarah, this is lovely. You made this?"

"Yes, I did. I learned how to knit from my grandmother, and I thought you might like this. I know it gets chilly in the evenings."

Mr. Thomas was touched by her thoughtfulness. "Thank you, Sarah. This means a lot to me."

As the years went by, Mr. Thomas and Sarah's friendship grew stronger. They would take walks together, go to the farmer's market on Saturdays, and even take trips to the beach. They were each other's confidants, and they knew they could always count on each other.

One day, Mr. Thomas fell ill. Sarah took care of him, cooking him meals and making sure he took his medicine. She visited him every day, making sure he wasn't alone. And when he finally passed away, she was there by his side.

Sarah missed Mr. Thomas terribly after he was gone. But she knew that their friendship would live on, and that he would always hold a special place in her heart. She smiled as she looked at the scarf he had worn every day, knowing that his memory would stay with her forever.

The Surprise Visit

It was a typical Thursday morning in the small town of Millfield. The sun was shining, the birds were chirping, and the town was buzzing with activity. Mr. Johnson, an elderly man who had lived in Millfield for over 60 years, was sitting on his porch enjoying the morning breeze when he heard a knock on the door.

He opened the door to find a young woman standing on his doorstep. "Hello, Mr. Johnson," she said with a smile. "I'm Lucy, your granddaughter."

Mr. Johnson was stunned. He had lost touch with his daughter and had never met his grandchildren. He invited Lucy in and sat down with her on the porch.

Lucy told him that she had been researching her family history and had discovered that Mr. Johnson was her grandfather. She had driven all the way from New York City to meet him and learn more about her family.

Mr. Johnson was overwhelmed with emotion. He had always longed for a family, and now he had one. He spent the day showing Lucy around town, introducing her to his friends, and telling her stories about his life. They had lunch at the local diner and visited the town museum.

As the day went on, Mr. Johnson realized how much he had missed out on by not having a family. He had always been content with his simple life, but now he saw how much richer it could have been.

Lucy spent a few more days with her grandfather, and they bonded over their shared love of music and books. She promised to visit him again soon and to stay in touch.

Mr. Johnson felt a renewed sense of purpose in his life. He began volunteering at the local library and joined a book club. He made new friends and became more involved in the community.

Years passed, and Mr. Johnson and Lucy remained close. She visited him every year and brought her own children to meet their great-grandfather. Mr. Johnson cherished every moment he spent with his family, and he felt grateful for the surprise visit that had changed his life forever.

The Piano Lesson

Mrs. Thompson had always loved music, especially classical piano. She had taken lessons as a child but had never pursued it seriously. Now, at the age of 80, she found herself longing to play again.

One day, she was sitting on her porch when she heard the sound of piano music coming from the house next door. She closed her eyes and listened, letting the music wash over her. It was beautiful.

She walked over to the neighbor's house and knocked on the door. A young man answered, and she could see the piano in the living room behind him. "Excuse me," she said. "I couldn't help but hear your playing. It was lovely."

The young man smiled. "Thank you. I'm glad you enjoyed it."

Mrs. Thompson hesitated for a moment, then asked, "Would you be willing to give me a piano lesson?"

The young man's face lit up. "Of course! I'd be happy to."

And so, every week, Mrs. Thompson went to the young man's house for a piano lesson. She was a little rusty at first, but she soon found that the music came back to her easily. She practiced every day, and soon she was playing with confidence.

As she played, she felt a sense of joy and peace that she hadn't felt in years. The music filled her heart and lifted her spirits. She realized that it was never too late to pursue a dream.

One day, the young man told her that he was moving away to attend music school. Mrs. Thompson was sad to see him go, but she was grateful for the time they had spent together.

She continued to play the piano every day, and her skills improved with each passing week. She began playing at local events and even gave a few concerts. People were amazed by her talent and her passion for music.

Mrs. Thompson felt alive again, as if a part of her had been awakened. She was grateful for the young man who had given her a chance to rediscover her love of music, and she knew that he would always hold a special place in her heart.

Years went by, and Mrs. Thompson passed away at the age of 90. At her funeral, a young woman stood up to play a beautiful piece on the piano. It was the young man's daughter, and she had learned the piece from her father, who had never forgotten the kind old woman who had inspired him to share his   love   of   music.

The Colorful Adventures of Mrs. Johnson

Mrs. Johnson was a sprightly old lady with a twinkle in her eye and a zest for life that never faded. She lived in a cozy little house in a quiet neighborhood, where she spent her days tending to her garden, reading her favorite books, and reminiscing about the colorful adventures of her youth.

One day, while browsing through her old photo album, Mrs. Johnson stumbled upon a snapshot that brought back a flood of memories. It was a picture of her and her childhood friends, all dressed up in their finest clothes, ready to embark on a grand adventure.

With a smile on her face and a skip in her step, Mrs. Johnson set out to reconnect with her old friends and relive the magic of their youthful adventures. She called each of them up and arranged a grand reunion, complete with a day trip to their favorite childhood haunt.

As they wandered through the streets of their old hometown, Mrs. Johnson and her friends marveled at the sights and sounds that had once been so familiar to them. They laughed and chatted, reminiscing about the days when they were young and carefree, and reliving the adventures that had shaped their lives.

They visited the old soda fountain where they used to hang out after school, and indulged in their favorite ice cream flavors. They strolled through the park, marveling at the beauty of the trees and flowers, and listening to the sound of the birds chirping in the trees.

As the day wore on, Mrs. Johnson and her friends grew tired but happy. They returned to Mrs. Johnson's house, where they sat around the table and shared stories over a hot cup of tea. They talked about their families, their careers, and the ups and downs of their lives.

As the sun began to set, Mrs. Johnson's friends bid her goodbye, promising to stay in touch and plan another adventure soon. Mrs. Johnson watched them go with a sense of contentment and joy in her heart, grateful for the memories they had shared and the sense of camaraderie that still bound them together.

As she settled into her favorite armchair, Mrs. Johnson smiled to herself and whispered a quiet prayer of thanks. She knew that the colorful adventures of her youth may be long gone, but the memories and friendships they had created would stay with her forever, a reminder of the beauty and joy of life that never fades.

The Magic of a Little Red Bicycle

Mr. Wilbur had always been a man who liked to take things slow. In fact, most people in his town thought of him as a bit of an oddball. He had never married, had no children, and spent most of his time pottering around his garden or tinkering with his old bicycle.

But Mr. Wilbur was happy with his quiet life. He didn't need anyone else to make him happy. That was until one day, he found a little red bicycle lying abandoned on the side of the road.

At first, Mr. Wilbur was hesitant to take the bike. It looked old and worn, and he wasn't sure if it would even work. But there was something about the way the sunlight glinted off the bike's shiny red paint that called out to him.

So, he took the bike home and spent the next few days fixing it up. He replaced the tires, oiled the chain, and even gave it a new coat of paint. And when he was done, the little red bicycle looked as good as new.

As soon as he hopped on the bike and started

pedaling, Mr. Wilbur felt like a young boy again. He pedaled down the road, the wind in his hair and the sun on his face. He felt free, like nothing in the world could hold him back.

But it wasn't until he rode the little red bicycle into town that things really started to change. People who had never spoken to him before started waving and saying hello. Children would run up to him and ask to see the bike. And as he rode around town, Mr. Wilbur found himself feeling more alive than he had in years.

One day, as he was riding past the local retirement home, he saw an elderly woman sitting alone on a bench. She looked sad and lonely, and Mr. Wilbur felt a pang of sympathy for her. So, he rode over to her and struck up a conversation.

Her name was Edith, and she had been living at the retirement home for the past few years. She told Mr. Wilbur about her life, and he listened intently, nodding and smiling as she spoke.

As they talked, Mr. Wilbur couldn't help but notice the way her eyes lit up when she talked about her childhood. She told him about growing up on a farm, riding horses, and playing with her siblings.

Suddenly, Mr. Wilbur had an idea. "Do you want to take a ride on my bike?" he asked.

Edith looked surprised but then nodded eagerly. Mr. Wilbur helped her onto the bike, and they pedaled off down the road, with the wind in their hair and the sun on their faces.

For the next few weeks, Mr. Wilbur and Edith became inseparable. They would ride around town on the little red bicycle, stopping to chat with friends and strangers alike. And every time they rode, Edith would talk about her childhood, and Mr. Wilbur would listen, feeling like he was learning more about life than he ever had before.

Eventually, the time came for Edith to leave the retirement home and move in with her daughter. Mr. Wilbur was sad to see her go, but he knew that they would always be friends.

As he rode home on the little red bicycle, Mr. Wilbur realized that he had found something he never knew he was missing. He had found joy in connecting with others, in learning from their experiences, and in sharing his own. And he knew that he had the little red bicycle to thank for it all.

The Rainbow Connection

It was a warm, sunny day in the small town of Millville, and the locals were out and about, enjoying the beautiful weather. Among them was a young girl named Lily, who was visiting her grandmother for the weekend.

As they strolled through the town, Lily's grandmother pointed out all of the sights and sounds, from the colorful flowers in the park to the sound of the church bells ringing in the distance. Lily was fascinated by it all and couldn't wait to explore more.

As they walked, they came across an old bookstore with a sign that read "Grand Opening." Intrigued, they decided to check it out. Inside, they were greeted by the owner, an older gentleman with a warm smile.

He welcomed them and showed them around the store, which was filled with books of every kind. Lily was in heaven, and her grandmother was thrilled to see her so excited.

The owner noticed Lily's enthusiasm and asked

her if she'd like to hear a story. Lily eagerly nodded, and the owner led them to a cozy corner of the store.

He began to tell them a tale of a young girl who loved to explore the world around her. She was fascinated by all the colors and sounds, and she loved to take in the beauty of the world. One day, she came across a rainbow in the sky, and she knew that it was a sign of hope and happiness.

As the owner spoke, Lily's grandmother couldn't help but feel nostalgic. She remembered all of the colors and sights and sounds of her own youth, and she was grateful for this moment with her granddaughter.

When the story was over, Lily was beaming with joy, and her grandmother felt uplifted and content. As they left the store, they looked up at the sky and saw a beautiful rainbow in the distance.

Lily's grandmother squeezed her hand and whispered, "Remember, my dear, that there's always something beautiful to look forward to."

And with that, they continued their stroll through the town, feeling grateful for the small moments that make life so wonderful.

The Colorful Surprise

It was a warm summer evening in the small town of Appleton, where the trees danced gently in the breeze, and the sweet scent of blooming flowers filled the air. At the center of town sat a little ice cream shop, where young and old alike gathered to enjoy the delicious flavors and refreshing treats.

Among the regular customers was an old man named Charlie, who had been coming to the ice cream shop for as long as he could remember. He loved the sweet and creamy flavors, but what he loved most was the sense of community and friendship that surrounded the place.

One day, as he was enjoying his usual scoop of vanilla ice cream, Charlie noticed something strange. The colors of the ice cream had changed. Instead of the usual plain vanilla, there were swirls of blue, green, and red mixed in.

He asked the young man behind the counter about it, who explained that they had a new flavor called Rainbow Swirl, which was a mix of different fruity flavors.

Charlie decided to give it a try and was pleasantly surprised by the burst of flavors in his mouth. As he savored the taste, memories flooded back to him of his childhood, when he used to pick berries from his grandmother's garden and make his own fruity ice cream.

Feeling nostalgic, Charlie struck up a conversation with the young man behind the counter, asking him about his life and dreams. The young man, whose name was Sam, shared his aspirations of becoming an artist and traveling the world.

Charlie encouraged Sam to pursue his dreams and reminded him that life is too short to not follow your passions. Sam was grateful for Charlie's kind words and the two of them continued to chat and share stories late into the evening.

As Charlie left the ice cream shop that night, he felt uplifted and grateful for the unexpected and colorful surprise that had brought him closer to a new friend. He realized that life is full of surprises and that every moment is an opportunity to make a connection and create a new memory.

From that day on, Charlie made it a point to try new flavors and strike up conversations with the young people he met. He discovered that they had much to teach him about the world and that he could still learn and grow, no matter how old he was.

And so, in the small town of Appleton, the ice cream shop became a place of not just sweet treats, but also of friendship, inspiration, and colorful surprises.

The Colorful Journey

The old man sat on his porch, gazing at the colorful sunset in the distance. His mind wandered back to his youth, a time when he lived a carefree life filled with adventure and excitement. As he reminisced, a young boy walked past, kicking a soccer ball with a sense of freedom and abandon.

"Hey there, son," the old man called out. "What brings you such joy?"

The boy stopped and looked up, a smile spreading across his face. "Just playing, sir. It's a beautiful day, isn't it?"

The old man nodded, taking in the sounds of children laughing and playing in the park. "Yes, it is. You know, I once had an adventure that took me to the most colorful places you could ever imagine."

The boy's eyes widened in excitement. "Really? Tell me about it!"

The old man leaned forward, his eyes sparkling with memories. "It all started when I was your age, just a young lad filled with curiosity and wonder. I remember walking down the street one day, when I heard the sound of a trumpet playing in the distance. I followed the sound, and before I knew it, I was at a carnival!"

The boy's face lit up with excitement. "A carnival! What did you see there?"

The old man's eyes glazed over, lost in memories. "Oh, everything! There were clowns with red noses and floppy shoes, acrobats flipping and twirling in the air, and games with prizes that shone like gold. But the most amazing thing of all was the carousel."

"The carousel?" the boy asked, intrigued.

The old man nodded, a smile spreading across his face. "Yes, the carousel. It was the most beautiful thing I'd ever seen, with horses and unicorns painted in every color of the rainbow. And when it started to spin, it was like I was transported to another world. The wind in my hair, the music in my ears, and the colors swirling around me – it was pure magic."

The boy grinned from ear to ear. "I want to go on a carousel like that one day!"

The old man chuckled. "I'm sure you will, son.

But remember, the most important thing is to never lose your sense of wonder. Life is full of adventures, big and small, and every one of them is worth experiencing with all your heart."

The boy nodded, taking in the old man's words. "Thank you, sir. I won't forget."

As the boy ran off to continue his game, the old man leaned back in his chair, his heart full of joy. It was true, he thought to himself – life was full of adventures, and he was grateful for every one of them. He closed his eyes, his mind filled with the sounds, sights, and colors of his colorful journey, and smiled contentedly.

The Colorful Carousel

Maggie sat on the park bench, staring at the colorful carousel that spun around and around, her heart aching with memories of her childhood. It had been so long since she had felt the excitement of the fairgrounds, the sweet scent of cotton candy, and the sound of laughter filling the air.

As she sat there lost in thought, a young boy sat down beside her, his eyes lighting up as he gazed at the carousel. "Isn't it beautiful?" he said.

Maggie smiled, "Yes, it is."

The boy asked, "Did you ride it when you were little?"

Maggie chuckled, "Oh, yes. I rode it many times."

The boy's eyes widened with wonder, "What was it like?"

Maggie closed her eyes, letting the memories flood back. "It was magical. The music played, and the horses galloped up and down. The colors were so bright and vivid, and the wind in my hair made me feel like I was flying."

The boy's face lit up with excitement, "Can we ride it together?"

Maggie hesitated for a moment, but then she smiled, "Sure, let's go."

They walked over to the carousel, and as they climbed onto the horses, Maggie felt a sense of joy she hadn't felt in years. The music started, and the horses began to move, up and down, around and around.

The boy laughed with delight, "This is amazing!"

Maggie felt tears prick at the corners of her eyes as she watched the boy's joy, feeling a deep sense of gratitude for this moment of happiness.

As the ride came to an end, they hopped off the horses, and the boy hugged Maggie, "Thank you, that was so much fun!"

Maggie smiled, "No, thank you. You reminded me of something I had forgotten, the joy of living in the moment and the beauty of life."

As they walked away, Maggie knew that she

would never forget the joy of the carousel, the sound of the music, and the colors of the horses, and most importantly, the happiness that came from sharing a moment of joy with someone else.

And as she walked away, she felt her heart filled with warmth and gratitude, knowing that even in the midst of life's challenges, there was always something to be grateful for, something to bring a smile to your face and light to your heart.

The Gift of Friendship

Mrs. Mary sat on her porch, rocking in her chair and watching the world go by. She had lived in the same house for over fifty years, and she had seen many changes in the neighborhood over the years. But one thing that had remained constant was her friendship with Mrs. Johnson.

Mrs. Johnson had been her neighbor for as long as she could remember, and they had grown old together, sharing the ups and downs of life. Mrs. Mary smiled as she thought about their daily walks, their tea times, and their long conversations about life, love, and everything in between.

One day, Mrs. Johnson had a stroke, and Mrs. Mary was devastated. She sat by her friend's bedside, holding her hand and praying for her to recover. But as the days turned into weeks, Mrs. Johnson's condition worsened, and Mrs. Mary feared the worst.

One day, as she sat by Mrs. Johnson's bedside, she realized that her friend was trying to say something. She leaned closer, listening carefully as Mrs. Johnson whispered, "Thank you for being my friend."

Mrs. Mary felt tears well up in her eyes, "You're my friend too, always."

As Mrs. Johnson slipped away, Mrs. Mary felt a deep sense of loss. But as she looked back on their years of friendship, she realized that the greatest gift she had ever received was the gift of Mrs. Johnson's friendship.

Years passed, and Mrs. Mary grew older. She often thought about her dear friend and the memories they had shared. One day, as she sat on her porch, a young girl walked up to her and smiled.

"Hello, Mrs. Mary. My name is Emily, and I'm your new neighbor."

Mrs. Mary smiled, "Hello, Emily. Welcome to the neighborhood."

As they talked, Mrs. Mary realized that she had found a new friend, someone to share her memories with, someone to walk with, and someone to talk to. And as she watched Emily walk away, she knew that her friendship with Mrs. Johnson had been a gift that had kept on giving, inspiring her to share her love, her wisdom, and her life with others.

As the sun set on the neighborhood, Mrs. Mary closed her eyes and felt a sense of peace, knowing that even in the midst of life's challenges, there was always something to be grateful for, something to bring a smile to your face and light to your heart.

The Magic of Music

Mr. Harold sat in his favorite armchair, listening to his old records and remembering the good old days. He had always loved music, and over the years, he had amassed a large collection of vinyl records, each one a treasure trove of memories.

As he listened to the music, he closed his eyes and let himself be transported back in time. He remembered his days in the army, where he had played trumpet in the band. He remembered his first dance with his wife, where they had danced to a slow song that had made his heart skip a beat.

He remembered the jazz clubs he used to go to with his friends, the sound of the saxophone, and the beat of the drums. He remembered the joy he felt every time he picked up his trumpet and played a few notes, the feeling of the music coursing through his veins.

As the music played, Mr. Harold felt a sense of joy and nostalgia wash over him. He realized that music was more than just entertainment; it was a way of life, a way of expressing emotions, and a way of connecting with others.

One day, he decided to share his love of music with his community. He contacted the local community center and offered to teach music lessons to anyone who wanted to learn. To his surprise, dozens of people showed up, eager to learn how to play an instrument or sing a song.

Mr. Harold was delighted to share his knowledge and experience with others, to see the joy on their faces as they discovered the magic of music. He watched as young children learned to play the piano, as teenagers formed a rock band, and as seniors rediscovered their love of singing.

As the years went by, Mr. Harold continued to teach music, and his community center became a hub of creativity and joy. People of all ages and backgrounds came together, united by their love of music.

And as Mr. Harold sat in his armchair, listening to the sounds of his community center echoing through the air, he felt a deep sense of pride and fulfillment. He had found his purpose in life, to share the gift of music with others, to spread joy and happiness, and to keep the magic of music alive for generations to come.

The Joy of Gardening

Mrs. Edith had always loved gardening. She had spent years cultivating her backyard, planting flowers, fruits, and vegetables. She loved the feel of the earth between her fingers, the sound of the birds singing, and the smell of the fresh soil.

Over the years, her garden had become her sanctuary, a place where she could escape the stresses of everyday life and immerse herself in the beauty of nature. She loved nothing more than watching her plants grow, seeing the colors of the flowers change with the seasons, and tasting the fresh produce straight from the garden.

As she grew older, however, Mrs. Edith found it harder to tend to her garden. Her back ached, and her hands were not as nimble as they used to be. She began to worry that she would have to give up her beloved garden.

One day, a group of teenagers from the local high school showed up at her doorstep. They were part of a community service program, and they offered to help Mrs. Edith tend to her garden.

Mrs. Edith was overjoyed. She had never expected anyone to offer to help her, and she was grateful for the young people's kindness. She showed them around her garden, explaining the different plants and their care.

The teenagers listened attentively, eager to learn from Mrs. Edith's wisdom and experience. They worked tirelessly, pulling weeds, watering the plants, and pruning the bushes. Mrs. Edith watched with delight as her garden began to thrive once again.

As the days went by, Mrs. Edith grew closer to the teenagers. She learned about their hopes and dreams, their struggles and successes. She shared stories from her own life, and the teenagers listened with rapt attention.

Together, they worked to create a beautiful and thriving garden, one that brought joy and happiness to Mrs. Edith and her community. And as she sat in her garden, surrounded by the beauty of nature and the warmth of friendship, Mrs. Edith knew that she had found a new purpose in life, to share her love of gardening with others, to inspire the next generation of gardeners, and to spread joy and happiness through the beauty of nature.

The Golden Train

Mrs. Winifred Adams was a sprightly lady of seventy-five who had lived her entire life in the small town of Millfield. She had a curious mind and a warm heart, and was loved by everyone in the town. She spent her days reading books, tending to her garden, and baking cakes for her friends and neighbors. But there was one thing she had always wanted to do - take a train journey across the country.

One day, while she was sitting in her garden, she heard a distant whistle. She knew it was the sound of a train, and it set her heart racing. She stood up and walked to the edge of her garden, and there it was - a gleaming golden train, snaking its way through the fields. She had never seen anything like it before. The train stopped at the station in Millfield, and Mrs. Adams knew that this was her chance.

She packed a small bag with some clothes, a few books, and some snacks, and headed to the station.

As she stepped onto the platform, she saw a young man who looked lost and confused. His name was Jack, and he was trying to find his way to his grandmother's house in another town. Mrs. Adams offered to help him, and they struck up a conversation.

As they chatted, Mrs. Adams found out that Jack was a musician. He had played the guitar since he was a young boy, and had always dreamed of making it big. But he had never had the courage to pursue his dream, and had settled for a job at a local store. Mrs. Adams listened to his story, and felt a pang of sadness in her heart. She knew what it was like to have unfulfilled dreams.

They boarded the train together, and found seats next to each other. As the train pulled out of the station, Mrs. Adams looked out of the window, and saw the world rushing by. The fields, the forests, the mountains, and the rivers - they all seemed to blur into one, like a colorful painting.

As they traveled across the country, Mrs. Adams and Jack met a host of interesting characters - a farmer who talked about his love for the land, a young couple who were on their honeymoon, and an old lady who had lived through two world wars. Each person had a story to tell, and Mrs. Adams listened to them all with rapt attention.

As the sun set on the first day of their journey, Mrs. Adams and Jack sat in the dining car, savoring a delicious meal. Jack took out his guitar and started playing a tune. It was a song he had written himself, and it was beautiful. Mrs. Adams closed her eyes and listened, and it brought tears to her eyes. She felt a surge of emotion, and realized that this was what it was like to live life to the fullest - to chase your dreams and to experience everything the world had to offer.

The next morning, as they neared their destination, Mrs. Adams and Jack said their goodbyes. Jack thanked her for the help she had given him, and for the friendship they had formed. Mrs. Adams hugged him tightly, and wished him all the best for his future. As she stepped off the train, she felt a sense of joy and contentment that she had never felt before. She had taken a chance, and it had paid off. She had made new friends, seen new places, and learned new things. She had lived.

As she walked to her home, Mrs. Adams looked up at the sky, and saw the sun shining brightly. It was a new day, and she knew that there were many more adventures waiting for her. She smiled, and whispered   to   herself,

The Colorful Treasure Hunt

It was a beautiful day in the small town of Springville, where the sun was shining bright, the birds were chirping, and the flowers were blooming. Mary, a young girl with a heart full of joy, was walking down the street with her grandmother, Emily, who was wise and kind. They were on a mission to find a treasure hidden somewhere in the town, which they heard about from the old folks at the nursing home.

As they walked, Mary couldn't help but admire the beauty of the town, with its colorful buildings, green parks, and the sound of the river flowing nearby. She could smell the fresh scent of flowers, and the taste of the sweetest ice cream she had ever tasted, which they bought from the local ice cream shop.

As they were enjoying their ice cream, they met an old man named Henry, who was sitting on a bench nearby. He overheard their conversation about the treasure hunt and offered to help them find it. Emily, being the wise one, welcomed his offer and they continued their journey together.

As they walked, they talked and laughed, and Mary learned about Henry's past, his adventures, and the lessons he learned throughout his life. He shared with her his love for painting, and how he always tried to capture the beauty of the world in his artwork. Mary was fascinated by his stories, and she couldn't wait to hear more.

As they reached the park, they saw a group of kids playing and laughing, and Emily had an idea. She suggested that they ask the kids to join their treasure hunt, and they happily agreed.

They followed the clues, and as they searched, they discovered the beauty of the town, the vibrant colors, and the different scents and sounds that surrounded them. Mary felt alive, and she knew that this was a day she would never forget.

Finally, they reached the end of their treasure hunt, and they found a chest full of gold coins. But that wasn't the real treasure. The real treasure was the memories they made together, the new friends they met, and the lessons they learned from each other.

As they sat on a bench, watching the sunset, Mary looked at Emily and Henry and realized that life is not about the things we have, but the people we love and the memories we create with them.

And as they walked back to the nursing home, Mary felt a sense of gratitude and joy in her heart, knowing that she had just experienced the most colorful treasure hunt of her life.

The Sweetest Surprise

As the sun began to rise over the small town of Cedarville, Mr. Harold Smith sat on his porch, enjoying his morning cup of coffee. Mr. Smith had lived in Cedarville for most of his life, and he knew everyone in the town. But lately, he had been feeling lonely. His children had grown up and moved away, and his wife had passed away years ago. He missed the companionship of a friend.

One day, as Mr. Smith was walking through town, he stumbled upon a little bakery he had never noticed before. The smell of freshly baked bread and pastries filled the air, and his mouth watered at the sight of the delectable treats in the display case.

As he walked in, he was greeted by the friendly face of a young girl named Emily. She welcomed him with a warm smile and introduced herself as the owner of the bakery. Mr. Smith couldn't help but notice the bright red apron she wore, which matched the red highlights in her curly brown hair. He was immediately charmed by her energy and enthusiasm.

Emily invited him to sit down at a small table and offered him a cup of coffee and a freshly baked cinnamon roll. As Mr. Smith savored the sweet, warm pastry, he couldn't help but feel a sense of happiness that he hadn't felt in a long time.

Over the next few weeks, Mr. Smith became a regular at the bakery. He would sit at the same table every day, sipping his coffee and chatting with Emily about everything from the weather to their favorite books. Emily would share stories about her own life, and Mr. Smith found himself feeling inspired by her optimism and resilience.

One day, as Mr. Smith was leaving the bakery, Emily handed him a small package. "This is for you," she said, her eyes twinkling with excitement.

When he opened the package, he found a beautifully decorated box of homemade chocolates. The sweet aroma of chocolate filled his nostrils, and his mouth watered at the sight of the various shapes and flavors.

Overwhelmed with gratitude, Mr. Smith hugged Emily tightly. "You have no idea what this means to me," he said, tears streaming down his face.

Emily smiled and hugged him back. "I know," she said softly. "That's why I did it."

From that day on, Mr. Smith felt a renewed sense of purpose and joy. He had found a friend in Emily, and their daily conversations filled his life with color and vitality. And every time he visited the bakery, he couldn't help but smile as he remembered the sweet surprise that had brought them together.

The Rainbow in the Garden

The sun was setting over the garden, casting a warm glow over the colorful flowers and green leaves. Old man Joe sat on a bench in the garden, lost in thought. His mind wandered back to his childhood, when he used to play in his grandmother's garden.

He remembered the sweet smell of the roses, the cool shade of the apple tree, and the sound of the birds singing. He closed his eyes and took a deep breath, reliving those memories.

Suddenly, he heard a voice calling out to him. "Hey there, old-timer! What are you doing all alone in the garden?" It was a young girl, no older than eight or nine, with bright red hair and a toothy grin.

Joe smiled at her and replied, "Just enjoying the beauty of nature, young lady. What brings you here?"

The girl plopped down on the bench next to him

and said, "I come here to watch the rainbow." Joe raised an eyebrow in surprise. "Rainbow? What rainbow?"

The girl pointed to a small fountain in the middle of the garden. "Every evening, when the sun sets just right, the water from the fountain sprays into the air and creates a rainbow. It's the most beautiful thing I've ever seen!"

Joe looked at the fountain, and sure enough, there was a faint rainbow hovering over it. He couldn't believe he had never noticed it before. The girl continued, "I come here every day to see the rainbow. It reminds me that there is still beauty in the world, even when everything seems dark and gloomy."

Joe felt a lump in his throat. He had been feeling down lately, and the girl's words touched him deeply. He looked at her with newfound respect and admiration. "You are a wise young lady," he said. "Thank you for reminding me of the beauty in the world."

The girl beamed at him. "You're welcome, sir! My name is Lily, by the way." Joe introduced himself, and they spent the next hour chatting and laughing.

As the sun set and the rainbow faded away, Joe felt a sense of happiness and contentment wash over him. He realized that he didn't have to be alone in his memories; he could make new ones with people of all ages.

He walked out of the garden, feeling lighter and more alive than he had in weeks. The world seemed a little brighter, a little more colorful, and a little more beautiful. And he knew that he had Lily to thank for that.

From that day on, Joe made it a point to visit the garden every evening, to watch the rainbow and to spend time with Lily. And every time he saw the rainbow, he felt a sense of hope and wonder, knowing that there was still magic in the world.

The Sweetness of Summer

In the sleepy town of Willow Springs, there lived an old lady named Alice. She had spent most of her life in that town, and as the years went by, she found herself reminiscing about the summers of her youth.

One day, as she sat on her porch, she heard the sound of children playing in the distance. It brought back memories of carefree days spent playing with her friends in the park. She decided to take a walk and see where the noise was coming from.

As she walked down the street, she saw a group of children playing in the park. They were laughing and running around, chasing each other, and having a great time. Alice couldn't help but smile at the sight.

As she got closer, she noticed a young boy sitting on a bench by himself, looking sad. She went over to him and asked him what was wrong.

The boy told her that he had just moved to town and didn't know anyone. Alice could relate to the feeling of being alone in a new place, and so she offered to show him around and introduce him to some of her friends.

They walked around the town, and Alice showed him all the places she loved as a child. They stopped at the local ice cream shop, and Alice treated him to a cone. As they sat outside, enjoying their ice cream, Alice shared stories from her youth, and the boy listened intently.

After a while, they said their goodbyes, and the boy went home. Alice walked back to her porch, feeling a sense of happiness she hadn't felt in a long time. She realized that the sweetness of summer was not just in the sights and sounds of the season, but in the connections we make with others.

From that day on, Alice made it her mission to connect with others in her town. She started volunteering at the local senior center, where she met people from all walks of life. She also continued to make new friends with the younger generations.

As the years went by, Alice never forgot the joy she felt that summer day. She continued to live her life with a sense of purpose and connection, and it brought her happiness in ways she never thought possible.

The sweetness of summer may fade with time, but the memories and connections we make can last a lifetime.

The Golden Years

Mrs. O'Malley was a spunky, gray-haired lady who lived in a cozy little house at the end of a winding road. She loved nothing more than sitting on her front porch, sipping sweet tea and watching the world go by. Her neighbor, Tommy, was a young boy who loved to ride his bike up and down the road, stopping to chat with Mrs. O'Malley every time he passed by.

One sunny afternoon, Tommy arrived at Mrs. O'Malley's porch with a basket full of freshly picked strawberries. "I thought you might like these, Mrs. O'Malley," he said, handing her the basket. "They're the best ones I could find."

Mrs. O'Malley's eyes lit up with delight. "Why, thank you, Tommy! I haven't had fresh strawberries in ages. You're a real sweetheart."

Tommy smiled, feeling proud of himself for making Mrs. O'Malley happy. As they chatted, Mrs. O'Malley began to reminisce about her own childhood. She told Tommy about the wildflower fields that used to grow where their houses now stood, and the sound of the old train whistle that would echo through the hills every afternoon.

As she spoke, Tommy found himself transported back in time, imagining what the world must have looked and sounded like when Mrs. O'Malley was his age. He could almost smell the wildflowers and feel the sun on his face.

Their conversation soon turned to the future, and Mrs. O'Malley admitted that she was a little scared of what lay ahead. "I've lived a good life," she said, "but I don't know what's coming next. Sometimes it feels like everything's changing so fast, and I can't keep up."

Tommy listened thoughtfully, then said, "You know, Mrs. O'Malley, I don't think you have to worry about the future. You've got all these great memories to look back on, and that's what really matters. Plus, you've got me to bring you strawberries and keep you company."

Mrs. O'Malley smiled, feeling a warmth spread through her chest. "You're right, Tommy. I'm lucky to have you and all my memories. I guess the golden years really are golden, aren't they?"

Tommy nodded, and they sat together in comfortable silence for a few moments, enjoying the warmth of the sun and the quiet hum of the neighborhood. As he rode his bike back down the road, Tommy felt a sense of contentment and happiness that he couldn't quite explain. Maybe it was the joy of making Mrs. O'Malley's day, or the excitement of hearing her stories. Or maybe it was just the simple pleasure of being alive and surrounded by love.

As for Mrs. O'Malley, she savored her strawberries and watched the world go by, feeling grateful for the gift of a new day and the memories of all the ones that had come before.

The Magical Afternoon

It was a crisp autumn day in the small town of Cedarville, where the leaves were ablaze in hues of red, orange and gold. Mrs. Thompson sat on her front porch, taking in the sights and sounds of the season. She loved the way the cool breeze carried the sweet smell of freshly baked pies from the nearby bakery. It reminded her of her childhood, when her mother used to make apple pies that were the talk of the town.

As she sat there, lost in thought, she noticed a little boy walking down the street. He was wearing a bright yellow raincoat and was jumping in the puddles that had formed after the morning rain. Mrs. Thompson smiled at the sight and couldn't help but remember her own son when he was that age. He loved nothing more than playing in the rain and getting soaked to the bone.

Just then, the little boy looked up and saw Mrs. Thompson sitting on her porch. He ran up to her with a big smile on his face and said, "Hi, I'm

Tommy! What's your name?"

Mrs. Thompson smiled back and said, "My name is Emily. It's nice to meet you, Tommy."

Tommy looked up at the sky and said, "It's a great day for jumping in puddles, isn't it?"

Mrs. Thompson couldn't help but laugh at his enthusiasm. "It sure is," she said. "Would you like to sit with me and have some hot chocolate?"

Tommy's eyes widened with excitement, and he eagerly accepted her offer.

As they sat on the porch, sipping on hot chocolate and sharing stories, Mrs. Thompson couldn't help but feel a sense of joy and contentment. She was grateful for this moment and the opportunity to connect with someone from a different generation.

They talked about their favorite colors, their favorite foods, and their favorite memories. Mrs. Thompson shared stories of her childhood and Tommy listened intently, imagining himself in her shoes.

As the sun began to set and the sky turned pink

and purple, Mrs. Thompson realized that this afternoon had been magical. It had reminded her of the beauty and simplicity of life, and the importance of cherishing every moment.

As Tommy said his goodbyes and ran back home, Mrs. Thompson sat there, lost in thought. She knew that this was a memory she would hold onto forever, and that it would bring her joy and comfort on days when she needed it most.

In that moment, Mrs. Thompson felt alive and grateful for the small moments that make life worth living.

The Surprise Birthday Party

Mrs. Jenkins had always loved a good party. Even at the ripe age of 87, she still had a twinkle in her eye at the thought of balloons, cake, and presents. But this year, she wasn't sure if she was going to have a birthday party at all.

She lived in a retirement home, and although the staff was always kind and caring, she didn't have any close friends to celebrate with. She missed her family terribly, but they lived too far away to visit often.

As her birthday approached, Mrs. Jenkins couldn't help but feel a little down. She tried to cheer herself up by taking walks in the park and playing cards with some of the other residents, but nothing seemed to lift her spirits.

One afternoon, she was sitting in the courtyard, watching the birds flit from tree to tree, when she heard a commotion coming from inside the building. Curious, she made her way back to her room, and when she opened the door, she was greeted with a sight that took her breath away.

There, in the middle of her room, was a group of people she had never seen before. They were of all ages, from a little girl with pigtails to a man with a gray beard. They were laughing and talking and holding brightly wrapped presents.

"Surprise!" they shouted when they saw her. Mrs. Jenkins was so surprised that she couldn't even speak. But then, one of the younger women stepped forward and gave her a big hug.

"We heard it was your birthday, and we wanted to do something special for you," she said. "We're your neighbors, from down the hall."

Mrs. Jenkins couldn't believe it. She had been so focused on her own loneliness that she hadn't even noticed the people who lived just a few doors down.

The group spent the afternoon eating cake, playing games, and telling stories. Mrs. Jenkins was amazed at the range of experiences they had all had. The man with the gray beard had been a sailor in the Navy, and the little girl with pigtails was an aspiring ballerina.

As the sun began to set, Mrs. Jenkins felt a sense of happiness she hadn't felt in a long time. She realized that even though she was getting older, there was still so much joy and beauty in the world. And she had new friends to share it with.

As the group began to say their goodbyes, Mrs. Jenkins hugged each one of them tightly. She knew that this would be a birthday she would never forget.

Walking back to her room, Mrs. Jenkins felt a renewed sense of purpose. She couldn't wait to see what other surprises life had in store for her. And who knows? Maybe she would even plan a surprise party of her own one day.

The Great Escape of Mr. Macintosh

Mr. Macintosh had lived a long and full life, but as he aged, he found himself growing more and more forgetful. One day, he decided to break out of his nursing home and go on a grand adventure.

He donned his old fedora and trench coat, grabbed his walking stick, and crept out of the door, avoiding the watchful eyes of the nurses. He wandered through the streets, taking in the sights and sounds of the bustling city, feeling a sense of freedom he hadn't felt in years.

As he strolled down the street, he heard a faint sound in the distance. It was the sound of a saxophone, playing a jazzy tune. Mr. Macintosh followed the sound to a small jazz club, where he saw a group of young musicians playing their hearts out.

He approached the stage, tapping his walking stick to the beat of the music. The musicians looked up, surprised to see an old man in a fedora standing before them. But they welcomed him with open arms, inviting him to sit in and play along.

Mr. Macintosh hesitated at first, unsure if he could still play, but the music took hold of him and he found himself lost in the melody. The other musicians cheered him on, and soon he was playing like he never had before.

For that one magical night, Mr. Macintosh forgot all about his age and his troubles. He laughed, he danced, and he played his heart out. The young musicians looked up to him with awe and respect, amazed by his talent and his spirit.

When the night came to an end, Mr. Macintosh said his goodbyes and made his way back to the nursing home. But he knew that he would never forget the feeling of that night, the feeling of being alive and free.

From that day on, Mr. Macintosh made it a point to break out of the nursing home whenever he could, always in search of the next great adventure. And although his memory may have been fading, he never forgot the magic of that night, the night he played his heart out and felt truly alive.

The Grand Adventure of Mr. Wilfred and the Mysterious Trunk

Mr. Wilfred was a sprightly old man, full of wit and humor. Despite his advancing age, he refused to let his spirits wane. So, when he discovered a dusty old trunk in his attic, he was immediately intrigued. It had belonged to his grandfather, who had been an intrepid explorer in his day. Mr. Wilfred was determined to unravel the mystery of the trunk and embark on his own adventure.

He spent hours poring over the contents of the trunk, which included maps, old journals, and exotic souvenirs. As he traced his grandfather's footsteps across the globe, Mr. Wilfred's imagination was fired up. He could almost hear the roar of the ocean and smell the spices of the orient.

One day, he stumbled upon a particularly intriguing journal entry. It spoke of a lost city deep in the heart of the Amazon, where a treasure beyond measure lay hidden. Mr. Wilfred was thrilled. This was it! He would go on an adventure to find the lost city and its treasure.

So, he set off on his journey, armed with his

grandfather's map and a sense of excitement that he hadn't felt in years. He traveled across seas and through dense jungles, facing danger at every turn. But Mr. Wilfred was undeterred. He was on a quest, and nothing would stand in his way.

As he ventured deeper into the jungle, he encountered strange creatures and made new friends. He marveled at the vivid colors of the flora and fauna, and savored the tastes and smells of exotic fruits and spices. Every step of the way, he felt his mind and body come alive with renewed vigor.

Eventually, Mr. Wilfred reached the lost city. He was awestruck by its grandeur, and his heart leapt with anticipation as he searched for the treasure. It took him days to uncover it, but when he finally did, he was speechless. It was a glittering mound of gold and jewels, the likes of which he had never seen.

As he made his way back home, Mr. Wilfred couldn't help but feel a sense of pride and accomplishment. He had gone on an adventure of a lifetime and emerged victorious. But more than that, he had rekindled the spark of youth within him. He realized that life was still full of wonder and joy, and that there was no age limit to adventure.

And so, Mr. Wilfred returned home a changed man. He regaled his friends with tales of his exploits and showed them the treasure he had found. But more than that, he inspired them to seek out their own adventures, no matter their age or circumstance.

For Mr. Wilfred, the adventure had just begun. He was ready to take on the world once more, armed with a sense of purpose and a zest for life that would never fade.

The Last Great Adventure

Maggie had always been an adventurous woman. She had traveled the world, climbed mountains, and explored the depths of the ocean. But now, at 90 years old, her body was failing her, and she was confined to a nursing home.

Maggie refused to let her spirit be confined, however. She spent her days chatting with her fellow residents, reading books, and reminiscing about her many adventures.

One day, while chatting with her friend Harold, Maggie had an idea. "Harold, do you remember that old plane I used to fly?" she asked.

Harold nodded. "Of course, Maggie. You were always the most fearless pilot I ever knew."

Maggie grinned. "Well, I was thinking, why don't we take one last great adventure together? We'll fly that old plane one more time, just for old times' sake."

Harold's eyes widened. "Are you serious?"

Maggie nodded. "Deadly serious. And I've got just the place in mind."

Maggie spent the next few weeks planning their great adventure. She called in favors from old friends, scoured the internet for maps and weather reports, and even dug up her old flight logs from decades ago.

Finally, the day arrived. Harold and Maggie climbed into the cockpit of the old plane, and Maggie fired up the engine. The sound of the propeller was music to her ears, and she felt alive again for the first time in years.

They soared through the air, over mountains and valleys, past fields and forests. They flew over the ocean, feeling the salt spray on their faces and the wind in their hair.

As they landed the plane, Harold turned to Maggie with tears in his eyes. "That was the most incredible thing I've ever experienced," he said.

Maggie smiled. "I'm glad I could share it with you, Harold. This may be my last great adventure, but it was the best one yet."

As they walked back to the nursing home, Maggie

felt a sense of contentment wash over her. She knew that even though her body may be failing, her spirit would always be free.

The Bus Trip

Mrs. Wilson had never been one for adventure. She was content with her quiet life in the small town where she had lived for the past 40 years. But when she saw an ad for a bus trip to a nearby city, something inside her stirred.

The day of the trip arrived, and Mrs. Wilson found herself on a bus full of strangers. As they drove through the countryside, she marveled at the sights and sounds around her. The green fields, the rolling hills, and the chirping of birds all made her feel alive in a way she hadn't felt in years.

The bus stopped in a small town for lunch, and Mrs. Wilson decided to explore. She wandered down a side street and found a quaint little bakery. The smell of fresh bread and pastries wafted out onto the street, and Mrs. Wilson couldn't resist going inside.

The bakery was bustling with activity, and Mrs. Wilson struck up a conversation with the woman behind the counter. She learned that the woman had started the bakery as a way to share her love of baking with others, and Mrs. Wilson was struck by the woman's passion and enthusiasm.

As she sat at a table enjoying her pastry and coffee, Mrs. Wilson realized that she had been missing out on so much by staying in her small town all these years. She had forgotten how exciting and exhilarating it could be to explore new places and meet new people.

The bus ride back to her town seemed shorter than the ride there, as Mrs. Wilson was lost in thought about all the adventures she wanted to have in the future. When she arrived home, she felt more energized and alive than she had in years.

From that day on, Mrs. Wilson made a point to seek out new experiences and adventures, and she was grateful for that bus trip that had opened her eyes to the possibilities all around her.

The Last Adventure of Gracie and Harold

Gracie and Harold had been married for over 60 years. They were now in their 80s and spent most of their time reminiscing about the good old days. They had traveled the world, had many adventures, and now they longed for one last adventure.

One sunny morning, they woke up with a newfound determination to go on a road trip. They packed a few things, said goodbye to their children and grandchildren, and hit the open road.

Their first stop was a small town where they stumbled upon a local bakery. The smell of freshly baked bread and pastries filled their noses, and they decided to buy a loaf of bread and some pastries. As they sat down to eat, they struck up a conversation with the owner, a kind and funny woman named Beth.

Beth told them about a little-known tourist attraction nearby, a hidden gem that only locals knew about. Gracie and Harold were intrigued and decided to check it out.

They followed Beth's directions and arrived at a small beach surrounded by cliffs. The sand was golden, and the water was crystal clear. They had never seen anything like it. They spent the day basking in the sun, listening to the sound of the waves crashing against the shore.

As the sun began to set, Gracie and Harold sat on a bench overlooking the beach. They watched as the sun slowly dipped below the horizon, turning the sky shades of pink and orange.

"This has been the best day of my life," Harold said, his eyes misty.

Gracie smiled. "Me too, Harold. Me too."

As they made their way back to their car, they knew that this would be their last adventure. They were both tired, but their hearts were full of memories and happiness.

They arrived home to find their family waiting for them. They shared their stories, and everyone was amazed by the pictures they had taken and the memories they had made.

Gracie and Harold went to bed that night with a sense of contentment and happiness. They knew that this adventure had been the perfect way to end their journey together.

As they drifted off to sleep, Gracie whispered, "Harold, we may be old, but we're not dead yet. Let's plan our next adventure."

Harold chuckled. "You're right, Gracie. The world is still full of surprises, and we're not done exploring it yet."

And with that, they both fell asleep, dreaming of the adventures that were still to come.

The Miracle of Mrs. Pennyworth

Mrs. Pennyworth had lived in the same small town for her entire life. She was now in her 90s and spent most of her days knitting, reading, and watching the world go by from her front porch.

One summer day, she noticed a group of children playing in the park across the street. They were laughing, running, and having the time of their lives. Mrs. Pennyworth watched them for a while, feeling a twinge of nostalgia for her own childhood.

As the day went on, Mrs. Pennyworth noticed that one of the children, a little girl named Lily, was crying. Mrs. Pennyworth went over to see what was wrong and found out that Lily's family was moving away, and she didn't want to leave her friends behind.

Mrs. Pennyworth knew how it felt to leave everything behind and start over, and her heart went out to the little girl. She sat with her and listened to her story, offering her a shoulder to cry on and a listening ear.

As Lily's family packed up their belongings, Mrs.

Pennyworth came up with an idea. She had a box filled with old trinkets and toys from her own childhood, and she decided to give it to Lily as a farewell gift.

Lily's eyes lit up as she rummaged through the box. There were marbles, dolls, puzzles, and even a kaleidoscope. Mrs. Pennyworth explained each item, telling stories of her own childhood and the adventures she had with each toy.

Lily's tears dried up, and she couldn't stop smiling. She hugged Mrs. Pennyworth tightly, thanking her for the most amazing gift she had ever received.

Mrs. Pennyworth watched as Lily's family drove away, feeling a sense of joy and contentment. She realized that even at her age, she still had the power to make a difference in someone's life.

As the years went by, Mrs. Pennyworth continued to watch the world go by from her front porch. She watched as the town changed, and new families moved in. She never forgot the joy she felt when she saw Lily's smile that day.

One day, Mrs. Pennyworth passed away peacefully in her sleep. As her belongings were being sorted through, the box of old toys was discovered. It had been carefully packed away, untouched for years.

Lily, now a grown woman, was contacted and invited to come and collect the box. She sat on Mrs. Pennyworth's porch, looking through the old trinkets and toys, feeling a sense of nostalgia and love.

As she left, she knew that Mrs. Pennyworth's gift had been more than just a box of toys. It was a reminder of the kindness and love that still existed in the world, and the impact that one person could make on another's life.

The Magic Biscuit Tin

Mrs. Margaret was an old lady with a heart of gold. She had lived a long and fulfilling life, filled with laughter, love, and adventure. As she sat in her cozy armchair one afternoon, she found herself reminiscing about the past. She thought of all the good times she had spent with her friends, the wonderful places she had visited, and the delicious food she had tasted.

Suddenly, she remembered something that brought a smile to her face. It was a magical biscuit tin that her grandmother had given her when she was a little girl. The tin was no ordinary biscuit tin, for it had the power to transport her to any place and time she desired.

Mrs. Margaret jumped up from her chair and ran to her attic. She rummaged through boxes and bags until she finally found the tin, hidden away at the back of a shelf. She dusted it off and opened the lid, and as she did so, a warm, comforting smell wafted up from inside.

Without hesitation, Mrs. Margaret reached in and took a biscuit. As she bit into it, she closed her eyes and let the taste and texture flood her senses. It was like a burst of sunshine in her mouth, and she felt a surge of energy and excitement.

She closed the lid of the tin and focused her thoughts on her destination. She wanted to go back to her childhood, to the village where she grew up, to the old bakery where she used to buy biscuits from the kind old baker.

With a whoosh, Mrs. Margaret felt herself being lifted off the ground. The world around her spun and twisted, and when she opened her eyes, she found herself standing in front of the old bakery, just as she remembered it.

The smell of freshly baked bread and pastries filled her nostrils, and the sound of the baker's whistle echoed in her ears. She walked inside and was greeted by the familiar face of the old baker, who looked just as she remembered him.

Mrs. Margaret spent the day exploring the village, meeting old friends, and reliving fond memories. She visited her old school, the park where she used to play, and the church where she got married.

As the sun began to set, Mrs. Margaret felt a sense of contentment wash over her. She had traveled back in time, and for a brief moment, she had felt like a child again.

As she opened the tin and took one last biscuit, she realized that the magic wasn't in the tin at all. It was inside her, in the memories and experiences that had shaped her into the person she was today.

With a smile on her face and a warm feeling in her heart, Mrs. Margaret closed the tin and walked back into her cozy home. She knew that she would never forget the magic of that day, and that the biscuit tin would always hold a special place in her heart.

And with that, she settled back into her armchair, content in the knowledge that life was full of magic and wonder, no matter how old you were.

The Quest for the Perfect Pie

Mrs. Maggie Smith had always been known in her small town for her delicious pies. People would come from far and wide just to taste her pies, and many of them would ask for her secret recipe. But Mrs. Smith would always smile and say, "I just put a little bit of love in every pie."

One day, Mrs. Smith realized that she had never tried making a pie with all of the fruits that she loved the most. So, she decided to embark on a quest to create the perfect pie.

She set out to the local market to gather all the fruits she needed: sweet peaches, juicy apples, tart cherries, and tangy berries. She picked out the best ingredients, carefully weighing and measuring each one.

As she was walking back home, she met an old friend, Mr. Brown. He asked what she was up to, and she told him about her quest for the perfect pie. Mr. Brown smiled and said, "You know, Mrs. Smith, I've always believed that the secret ingredient in any great pie is a little bit of mischief."

Mrs. Smith was puzzled by Mr. Brown's comment, but she shrugged it off and continued her quest. She spent hours mixing, rolling, and baking her fruits into a delicious pie. Finally, it was ready.

She cut a slice and took a bite, but something was missing. She tried again and again, but it just wasn't the perfect pie she had been hoping for.

Just as she was about to give up, she remembered Mr. Brown's words about mischief. She decided to add a little bit of something extra to her pie, something she had never tried before.

With a mischievous glint in her eye, she added a pinch of cinnamon and a dash of nutmeg to her pie. She took a bite and closed her eyes. It was the most delicious pie she had ever tasted!

Mrs. Smith realized that Mr. Brown was right. Sometimes, adding a little bit of mischief to a recipe can make all the difference. She smiled to herself and thought, "I guess there's still some mischief left in this old lady yet!"

From that day on, Mrs. Smith continued to create new and delicious pies, always adding a little bit of mischief to each one. She became famous for her unique and delicious creations, and people would come from far and wide just to taste her pies.

And whenever she was asked for her secret recipe, she would just smile and say, "I put a little bit of love and a little bit of mischief in every pie."

The Great Lemonade Stand Caper

Old Mr. Jenkins was feeling blue. He had retired from his job as a schoolteacher years ago and had been spending his days in his rocking chair, feeling lonely and bored. He longed for the days when he used to take his students on adventures and make them laugh with his silly stories.

One day, as he was gazing out the window, he saw a group of kids setting up a lemonade stand on the sidewalk. They were shouting and laughing, and their colorful sign promised the best lemonade in town.

Mr. Jenkins felt a pang of nostalgia as he remembered how he used to help his students set up their own lemonade stands. He decided that he was going to pay the kids a visit.

When he arrived at the stand, the kids welcomed him with open arms. They offered him a cup of lemonade, and Mr. Jenkins was surprised at how delicious it was. He complimented the kids on their recipe, and they eagerly shared their secret ingredient: a pinch of cinnamon.

Mr. Jenkins was delighted. He realized that he had been missing the joy of teaching and learning from young minds. He offered to help the kids with their lemonade stand, and they gladly accepted.

Together, they brainstormed new flavors and even created a special recipe with fresh berries from Mr. Jenkins' garden. The lemonade stand became the talk of the town, and people came from far and wide to try their unique and delicious concoctions.

Mr. Jenkins felt his spirits lift as he spent his days with the kids, joking and laughing and learning new things. He realized that he didn't have to retire from life just because he retired from his job. He could still be a mentor and a friend to young people.

And so, Mr. Jenkins spent the rest of his days helping the kids with their lemonade stand, and they all became the best of friends.

The Adventures of Grandma Gertie

Grandma Gertie was a spunky old lady with a zest for life. At the age of 80, she still had the energy of someone half her age. She loved nothing more than going on adventures and exploring new places. Her favorite pastime was people-watching at the local park, where she would strike up conversations with anyone who crossed her path.

One sunny afternoon, Grandma Gertie was sitting on a park bench when she overheard two young girls talking about their upcoming camping trip. She couldn't resist chiming in and telling them about the time she went camping in the mountains with her husband many years ago. The girls were fascinated by her story and asked her to join them on their trip.

Grandma Gertie hesitated at first, but then decided to take them up on their offer. She dug out her old camping gear from the attic and packed her bags. The day of the trip arrived, and Grandma Gertie was ready for adventure.

The girls led her on a hike through the woods, pointing out all the different types of trees and animals they saw along the way. Grandma Gertie was amazed by the vibrant colors of the leaves and the sound of the birds chirping in the trees.

As they set up camp for the night, Grandma Gertie regaled the girls with stories of her youth. She told them about the time she won a pie-eating contest at the county fair and how she used to sneak out of the house to go dancing with her friends. The girls were captivated by her tales, and they all laughed and joked around the campfire.

During the night, a sudden rainstorm hit, and the girls were afraid they would have to pack up and leave. But Grandma Gertie had a trick up her sleeve. She pulled out a set of cards and taught the girls how to play a game of Go Fish. They played for hours, forgetting about the rain and enjoying each other's company.

The next morning, the rain had stopped, and the sun was shining once again. Grandma Gertie and the girls packed up their gear and hiked back to the park. As they said their goodbyes, the girls thanked Grandma Gertie for coming on the trip with them. Grandma Gertie smiled and told them that she had the time of her life.

From that day forward, Grandma Gertie made a

point of going on more adventures and meeting new people. She realized that no matter how old she got, there was always something new to discover and learn. And every time she went on an adventure, she felt more alive and energized than ever before.

The Misadventures of Mr. Jenkins

Mr. Jenkins was an elderly gentleman with a love for adventure. He spent his days wandering the streets of his town, taking in the sights and sounds around him. But on this particular day, Mr. Jenkins found himself on a wild adventure he never expected.

As he was walking down the street, he heard a commotion coming from a nearby alleyway. Curiosity getting the better of him, Mr. Jenkins ventured into the alley, where he found a group of mischievous children causing trouble. They were throwing rocks at a stray cat, and Mr. Jenkins knew he had to intervene.

With a stern voice, Mr. Jenkins scolded the children for their behavior and rescued the cat from their grasp. He held the cat close to his chest and felt its soft fur against his skin. The cat purred in his arms, and Mr. Jenkins knew he had made a new friend.

As he walked back home with the cat in tow, Mr. Jenkins noticed a peculiar smell coming from the alleyway. It was a smell he couldn't quite place, but it reminded him of something from his childhood. Suddenly, a flood of memories came rushing back to him.

He remembered his mother's homemade apple pie and the scent of fresh-cut grass in the summertime. He remembered the taste of ice cream on a hot day and the feeling of sand between his toes at the beach. Mr. Jenkins realized that the scent in the alleyway had triggered his memories and made him feel young again.

Over the next few days, Mr. Jenkins and the cat became inseparable. They went on adventures together, exploring new places and making new friends. Mr. Jenkins felt like a kid again, and he loved every minute of it.

But one day, the cat disappeared. Mr. Jenkins searched high and low for his furry friend but couldn't find her anywhere. He felt a pang of sadness in his heart, wondering if he would ever see her again.

Just as he was about to give up hope, the cat appeared out of nowhere, meowing loudly at his feet. Mr. Jenkins scooped her up into his arms, feeling the warmth of her body against his own. He knew that they would be together forever, exploring the world and creating new memories along the way.

As Mr. Jenkins walked back home, he realized that the adventures he had with the cat had brought him more joy and happiness than he had felt in years. And he knew that as long as he kept his sense of curiosity and wonder alive, there would always be more adventures waiting for him just around the corner.

The Great Adventure of Ms. Mildred and the Mischievous Grandkids

Ms. Mildred was an elderly woman who lived alone in a small cottage in the countryside. She had a passion for adventure and loved exploring new places, but age had taken its toll on her body, and she could no longer travel as she used to.

One day, Ms. Mildred's mischievous grandkids came to visit her. They were always up to some mischief and loved playing pranks on their grandma. However, Ms. Mildred had a surprise for them. She had discovered a hidden treasure map in her attic, which led to a mysterious island, where a legendary treasure was said to be hidden.

The grandkids were thrilled at the prospect of finding the treasure, and Ms. Mildred was excited to go on an adventure with her grandchildren. So, they packed their bags and set off on a journey to find the treasure.

As they journeyed, they encountered various challenges and obstacles. They had to cross a raging river, climb a steep mountain, and navigate through a dense forest. Along the way, they met many interesting characters, including a talking parrot who gave them clues about the treasure's location.

Despite the challenges, Ms. Mildred and her grandkids persevered and finally arrived at the island. They searched high and low for the treasure, but it was nowhere to be found. Just as they were about to give up, they stumbled upon an old chest hidden in a cave.

With trembling hands, Ms. Mildred opened the chest, and to her surprise, it was filled with old photographs, letters, and trinkets. As she sorted through the items, memories of her youth came flooding back. She shared stories of her past adventures with her grandkids, and they laughed and reminisced about old times.

In the end, Ms. Mildred realized that the treasure she had been searching for was not gold or jewels, but the memories and experiences she had shared with her family and loved ones.

As they journeyed back home, Ms. Mildred and her grandkids were exhausted but filled with joy and gratitude. They had created new memories together and strengthened their bond as a family.

The adventure may have come to an end, but the

memories and lessons they had learned would stay with them forever. Ms. Mildred and her grandkids hugged each other tightly, knowing that they had found the greatest treasure of all - the love and warmth of family.

The Secret Recipe

Mrs. Jenkins was a sprightly old lady who lived in a small town. She had always been known for her delicious baked goods, and her apple pie was the talk of the town. But as she grew older, her memory began to fail her, and she feared that her famous recipe would be lost forever.

One day, Mrs. Jenkins met a young girl named Lily, who was new in town. They struck up a conversation, and Mrs. Jenkins shared her love for baking with Lily. To her surprise, Lily also had a passion for baking and loved making cupcakes.

Mrs. Jenkins felt a spark of excitement and shared her secret apple pie recipe with Lily. She cautioned her not to share it with anyone else, as it was a family recipe that had been passed down through generations.

Lily was overjoyed at the thought of learning the secret recipe, and she promised to keep it safe. She spent hours perfecting the recipe and even added her own special twist to it.

Meanwhile, Mrs. Jenkins had forgotten that she

had shared the recipe with Lily and began to worry about it being lost forever. She went to great lengths to find the recipe, even checking in the most unusual places, but to no avail.

One day, Lily surprised Mrs. Jenkins with a freshly baked apple pie. The aroma filled the room, and Mrs. Jenkins' eyes lit up. She took a bite and closed her eyes, savoring the taste. It was the best apple pie she had ever tasted, and she knew that her secret recipe was in good hands.

Lily had not only perfected the recipe but had also added her own touch, which made it even better. Mrs. Jenkins was overjoyed and proud of Lily for keeping the recipe alive.

From that day on, Mrs. Jenkins and Lily became the town's baking duo. They baked and shared their creations with everyone in town, spreading joy and happiness wherever they went.

Mrs. Jenkins had realized that sharing her secret recipe had not only kept her memory alive but had also brought her closer to a new friend. Lily had learned the importance of keeping traditions alive and had also discovered a new passion.

As they baked together, Mrs. Jenkins and Lily

shared stories of their past and their hopes for the future. They laughed and bonded over their love for baking, and Mrs. Jenkins realized that her memory may have faded, but her love for baking and making new friends would never die.

The Sweetest Confection

Once upon a time, in a small town nestled in the heart of the countryside, there lived an elderly man named Henry. Henry was a retired candy maker who spent his days reminiscing about his sweetest confection, a candy that he had created long ago that had won him many awards.

Despite his age, Henry's mind was still sharp, and his memories of the candy-making process were as clear as day. He could recall the colors, sights, sounds, tastes, smells, and feelings that went into creating his masterpiece, and he longed to taste it again.

One day, a young woman named Lily came into Henry's candy shop. Lily was a budding confectioner who was fascinated by the art of candy making, and she wanted to learn all that she could from Henry.

Over the next few weeks, Lily and Henry worked together to create a new candy that would rival Henry's old masterpiece. They mixed and stirred, tasted and tested, until finally, they came up with a candy that was even sweeter than the original.

Henry was thrilled to taste the new candy and was surprised at how well Lily had managed to capture the essence of his old recipe. He was so pleased that he decided to share the candy with his friends at the local retirement home.

When they arrived at the retirement home, Henry and Lily were greeted by a group of eager residents, all excited to taste the new candy. As they passed around the candy, the residents' faces lit up with delight.

Henry was overjoyed to see the happiness that his candy had brought to his friends' lives, and he realized that he had found a new purpose in life. He and Lily continued to work together, creating new and exciting candies to share with the residents of the retirement home.

As time passed, Henry's candy shop became a gathering place for the young and old alike. It was a place where people could come and taste the sweetest confections and make new friends. Henry had found a new lease on life, and he was grateful for the joy that his candy had brought to so many.

In the end, Henry realized that the sweetest confection was not the candy itself, but the joy and happiness that it brought to others. He knew that as long as he had his candy and his friends, he would never be alone or bored, and he

could continue to create memories that would last a lifetime.

And so, Henry continued to create new candies and share them with his friends, both young and old. He had found a new purpose in life, and he was grateful for the opportunity to make a difference in the lives of those around him.

As for Lily, she had found a mentor and a friend in Henry. Together, they had created something truly special, and she knew that her life would never be the same.

And so, as the days turned into weeks, and the weeks turned into months, Henry's candy shop remained a place of joy, laughter, and friendship. And as for Henry himself, he was happy knowing that he had made a difference in the lives of those around him, and that his sweetest confection would continue to bring happiness to others for years to come.

The Great Adventure

In a small town in the middle of nowhere, there lived an elderly woman named Martha. She had lived in the town her whole life and had never ventured beyond its borders. She had always dreamed of traveling the world and experiencing new things, but she had never had the chance.

One day, Martha's granddaughter, Emily, came to visit. Emily had just returned from a trip around the world and had brought back stories of her adventures that filled Martha with excitement.

As they sat in Martha's garden, Emily shared stories of exotic lands, vibrant cultures, and fascinating people. She talked about the colors, sights, sounds, tastes, smells, and feelings that she had experienced on her journey, and Martha was captivated.

She realized that it wasn't too late to have an adventure of her own. She decided to pack her bags and set out to explore the world, with Emily as her guide.

Their first stop was Paris. Martha was amazed by

the city's beauty and charm. They visited the Eiffel Tower, the Louvre, and the Champs-Élysées. Martha tried French pastries and cheeses for the first time, and the flavors exploded in her mouth.

Next, they traveled to Tokyo. Martha was fascinated by the city's bustling streets and neon lights. They visited the temples and shrines, and Martha tried sushi for the first time. She was surprised by how much she enjoyed the taste of raw fish.

Their final stop was Rio de Janeiro. Martha was entranced by the city's vibrant colors and festive atmosphere. They visited the beaches and danced the samba. Martha tried caipirinhas and found them to be delicious.

As they made their way back home, Martha realized that she had not only fulfilled her dream of seeing the world but had also discovered new passions and interests. She had learned that it was never too late to try something new and that life was full of surprises.

Martha returned home feeling alive and rejuvenated. She had experienced the world in a way that she never thought possible, and she was grateful for the opportunity. She knew that she would never forget the sights, sounds, tastes, smells, and feelings of her great adventure.

And as for Emily, she was happy to have shared her love of travel with her grandmother and to have created memories that they would both cherish for the rest of their lives.

The Unlikely Friendship

Mrs. Pearl, an 85-year-old lady, loved to sit on her porch every morning and watch the world go by. She had lived in the same house for over 50 years and had seen a lot of changes in her neighborhood. She liked to reminisce about the old days when things were simpler.

One day, while Mrs. Pearl was sitting on her porch, she noticed a young man walking down the street. He looked lost, so she called out to him and asked if he needed any help. The man introduced himself as Tim and explained that he was new to the neighborhood and looking for a job.

Mrs. Pearl was intrigued by Tim's story, so she invited him to sit with her on the porch and talk. Tim was hesitant at first, but he could see the kindness in Mrs. Pearl's eyes and decided to stay.

As they sat and chatted, Mrs. Pearl learned that Tim was a struggling artist. He had moved to the city to pursue his dreams of becoming a famous painter, but so far, things had not gone as planned. Mrs. Pearl had always loved art, so she asked to see some of Tim's work.

Tim was hesitant to show her his paintings, but when he did, Mrs. Pearl was blown away. She saw so much life and color in his paintings, and she could tell that he had a real talent for art.

Over the next few weeks, Mrs. Pearl and Tim became good friends. They spent hours on the porch talking about art, music, and life. Mrs. Pearl even gave Tim some tips on how to sell his paintings and make a living as an artist.

One day, Tim surprised Mrs. Pearl with a painting he had done just for her. It was a beautiful portrait of her sitting on the porch, with the sun shining on her face and the flowers blooming around her. Mrs. Pearl was so touched by the painting that she started to cry.

From that day on, Mrs. Pearl and Tim became inseparable. They went on walks together, visited art galleries, and even took a painting class together. Mrs. Pearl's memory was stimulated by all the new experiences she was having with Tim, and her imagination was alive and well.

As for Tim, he was inspired by Mrs. Pearl's zest for life and her sense of humor. She had a way of making him feel good, even when things were tough.

In the end, Mrs. Pearl and Tim proved that age is just a number, and that unlikely friendships can be the best kind. They both learned a lot from each other, and their friendship kept them both young at heart.

The Adventure of Mr. Winston

Mr. Winston was an old man who had lived a long and fulfilling life. He had traveled the world, met many interesting people, and had more stories to tell than he could count. But as he grew older, he found himself spending more and more time alone. His body wasn't as spry as it used to be, and he couldn't do all the things he used to enjoy.

One day, Mr. Winston decided he needed a change of scenery. He packed his bags and set out on a journey to a small town in the countryside. He had heard that there was a magical garden there, filled with all sorts of exotic plants and flowers. He was determined to see it for himself.

When Mr. Winston arrived in the town, he was surprised to find that it was filled with young people. There were families with children running around, teenagers hanging out at the local cafe, and young couples strolling hand in hand. Mr. Winston felt a little out of place among all the youthful energy, but he decided to make the best of it.

He went to the local cafe and struck up a conversation with a group of teenagers. They were fascinated by his stories of traveling the world and meeting famous people. They asked him questions and listened with rapt attention as he regaled them with tales of adventure.

As he sat in the cafe, Mr. Winston realized that he wasn't as old as he thought he was. He may not have the same energy as the young people around him, but he still had a sharp mind and a wealth of experience. He decided to embrace his inner youth and see where it took him.

The next day, Mr. Winston set out to find the magical garden. He wandered through the town, taking in the sights and sounds around him. He stopped to smell the flowers in the local park and listened to the birds singing in the trees.

As he walked, Mr. Winston met a young woman named Lily. She was an aspiring artist who had moved to the town to escape the hustle and bustle of the city. They struck up a conversation, and Mr. Winston was impressed by her creativity and passion.

Together, they set out to find the magical garden. They walked for hours, through fields and forests, until they finally stumbled upon it. The garden was even more beautiful than Mr. Winston had imagined. There were flowers of every color and shape, and the air was filled with the scent of jasmine and lavender.

As they walked through the garden, Lily told Mr. Winston about her dreams of becoming a famous painter. He listened intently and offered her advice from his own experiences. She was grateful for his words of wisdom and felt inspired to pursue her dreams even more passionately.

As they left the garden, Mr. Winston felt a sense of contentment that he hadn't felt in a long time. He had made a new friend, helped her to find inspiration, and had discovered that age was just a number. He realized that there was still so much he could do, so much he could learn, and so much he could experience.

As he returned to his home, Mr. Winston felt a renewed sense of purpose. He was grateful for the adventure he had embarked on, and he knew that there were many more to come. He smiled himself, feeling young and alive once again.

The Golden Memories

Once upon a time, in a small town named Pleasantville, lived an old man named George. George was in his late 80s and had lived a long and fulfilling life. He loved to sit on his porch and watch the world go by. He had seen many things in his life, and he often reminisced about his past.

One day, while sitting on his porch, he saw a group of children playing in the street. They were laughing, screaming, and having the time of their lives. George couldn't help but smile as he watched them. He remembered his own childhood and all the adventures he had.

As he watched the children, he realized that he had not been having as much fun lately. He had been feeling down and lonely. He knew he needed to do something to lift his spirits.

George decided to take a walk through the town. As he walked, he saw familiar places that reminded him of his past. He saw the park where he used to play baseball, the bakery where he used to get his favorite apple pie, and the movie theater where he saw his first film.

As he was walking, he came across a young girl named Lily. She was selling lemonade on the street. George stopped to buy a cup, and they started talking. Lily told George about her dreams and aspirations. George shared some of his own stories, and they both laughed and smiled.

From that day on, George started to take walks every day. He met new people, made friends, and shared his stories. He realized that he had so much to give and that he could still make a difference in the world. He felt alive again.

One day, George was walking through the town square when he saw a flyer for a talent show. He decided to enter and share his love for music. He dusted off his old guitar, practiced for weeks, and finally performed in front of a large crowd. The audience cheered, and George felt like a rock star.

After the show, he was approached by a group of young musicians who wanted to start a band with him. George felt honored and excited. He never thought that he could still have such a meaningful impact on people's lives.

George realized that age was just a number. He learned that he could still learn new things, make friends, and have fun. He felt grateful for his life and all the memories he had made. He knew that he would continue to create new memories for as long as he lived.

And so, George's golden memories lived on, bringing joy and inspiration to everyone he met.

The Magnificent Cake Contest

Mrs. Beatrice had always been known for her exquisite baking skills. Her cakes were the talk of the town, and everyone who tasted them agreed that they were simply heavenly. But despite all the compliments, Mrs. Beatrice felt that something was missing in her life. She had been feeling lonely ever since her husband passed away, and she longed for some excitement and adventure.

One day, she saw an advertisement for a cake contest in the local newspaper. It was going to be a huge event, with participants from all over the state. The grand prize was a trip to Paris, and Mrs. Beatrice knew she had to enter. She spent weeks preparing her cake, carefully selecting the ingredients and mixing them with love and dedication.

On the day of the contest, Mrs. Beatrice was nervous but excited. She arrived at the venue, a grand ballroom decorated with colorful balloons and streamers. There were tables set up for each contestant, and the cakes on display were a sight to behold. Some were tall and elaborate, while others were simple and elegant.

As the judges made their rounds, tasting each cake and taking notes, Mrs. Beatrice's nerves began to dissipate. She struck up conversations with the other contestants, and soon they were sharing stories and laughter. She learned about their hometowns and their families, and even got some new baking tips.

Finally, the judges announced the winners. Mrs. Beatrice's heart was pounding as she listened to the names being called out. Third place went to a young woman who had made a vegan cake, second place went to a man who had used fresh fruits in his recipe, and then came the moment of truth. The first prize went to Mrs. Beatrice!

Tears of joy streamed down her face as she went up to collect her award. She hugged the judges and thanked them profusely, and then turned to face the cheering crowd. As she looked out, she saw familiar faces beaming with pride. Her children, grandchildren, and even great-grandchildren had come to see her win. They hugged her and told her how proud they were, and Mrs. Beatrice felt a warmth in her heart that she hadn't felt in a long time.

The trip to Paris was amazing, and Mrs. Beatrice

returned home with a newfound sense of purpose. She started baking more cakes, trying out new recipes and experimenting with flavors. She also started volunteering at a local nursing home, sharing her baking skills and stories with the elderly residents. She felt fulfilled and happy, and knew that the Magnificent Cake Contest had changed her life forever.

In the end, Mrs. Beatrice realized that life is full of surprises and adventures, no matter how old you are. All you need is a little courage and a lot of love, and anything is possible.

The Miracle of the Magic Garden

Mrs. Potts had always been a lover of nature. She spent her days tending to her garden, carefully pruning the flowers and shrubs and watching them bloom into a beautiful array of colors. Her garden was her sanctuary, her happy place, and she spent most of her time there.

One day, a young boy named Tommy wandered into her garden. He was fascinated by the beauty of the flowers and the sweet fragrance that filled the air. Mrs. Potts smiled at him and invited him to take a closer look. Tommy was delighted and spent the entire afternoon exploring the garden with Mrs. Potts.

As the sun began to set, Mrs. Potts realized that Tommy had missed his lunch. She took him inside and made him a delicious sandwich with fresh vegetables from her garden. Tommy ate heartily and thanked her for her kindness.

From that day on, Tommy became a regular visitor to Mrs. Potts' garden. They would spend hours talking about nature and life, and Tommy would help her with the gardening chores. Mrs.

Potts felt rejuvenated by his youthful energy and enthusiasm, and Tommy loved learning from her wisdom and experience.

One day, as they were sitting in the garden, Tommy noticed that one of the flowers was wilting. He asked Mrs. Potts what they could do to save it. She thought for a moment and then had an idea. She told Tommy that they needed to perform a magic ritual to bring the flower back to life.

Tommy was skeptical but intrigued. Mrs. Potts took out a small bottle of perfume and sprinkled a few drops on the flower. She then closed her eyes and whispered some words that Tommy couldn't understand. Suddenly, the flower began to bloom again, as if by magic.

Tommy was amazed and asked Mrs. Potts how she had done it. She smiled and told him that it was the Miracle of the Magic Garden. She explained that sometimes, all it takes is a little love and imagination to make things come alive.

Tommy was thrilled and asked Mrs. Potts if he could learn more about the magic of the garden. She agreed and they spent the rest of the summer exploring the mysteries of nature, learning about the healing powers of herbs and flowers, and discovering the joy of working together to create something beautiful.

As the days grew shorter and the air turned colder, Tommy knew that he would miss his time in the garden with Mrs. Potts. But he also knew that he would carry the magic of the garden with him wherever he went, and that it would keep his imagination alive and his mind active for years to come.

Mrs. Potts, too, felt a sense of fulfillment and joy. She realized that age was just a number, and that as long as she had her love of nature and her passion for life, anything was possible. She knew that the Miracle of the Magic Garden would stay with her forever, and that it would continue to bring joy and happiness to all who encountered it.

The Great Escape

It was a typical day at the retirement home, and Martha was feeling particularly restless. She had been living at the home for a few years now and had grown tired of the same old routine. She longed for something exciting, something that would make her heart race.

As she sat in the common room, staring out the window, she noticed a young man walking by outside. He was carrying a guitar and had a carefree look about him. Martha felt a pang of envy. She missed her youth, the days when she was free to roam and explore.

Suddenly, an idea struck her. What if she and some of her friends could escape the retirement home for a day of adventure? The thought of breaking the rules thrilled her.

Martha approached her friend Betty, who was always up for a good time. Betty was hesitant at first, but Martha convinced her that it was time for a little excitement. Together, they recruited a few more adventurous souls from the home, including a former pilot and a retired nurse.

The group hatched a plan. They would sneak out of the home after dinner and meet the young man with the guitar outside. He would take them on an adventure they would never forget.

As the sun set that evening, the group snuck out of the home and met the young man, whose name was Jake. He greeted them with a smile and led them to a nearby park.

The park was alive with color, sound, and activity. Children played on the swings, dogs chased each other around the grass, and a band played music on a nearby stage. The group was overjoyed at the sight of so much life.

They spent the evening listening to music, dancing, and laughing. They ate ice cream and hot dogs and drank lemonade. They shared stories of their youth and talked about their dreams for the future.

As the night wore on, Martha felt her spirits lifted. She realized that age was just a number and that there was still so much life left to live. She felt young again, and she knew that her fellow adventurers felt the same.

Eventually, it was time to return to the retirement home. The group said goodbye to Jake and promised to keep in touch. Martha and her friends returned to their rooms, exhausted but exhilarated.

The next day, Martha woke up feeling energized. She had a renewed sense of purpose and a newfound appreciation for life. She knew that she would never forget the great escape she had shared with her friends, and she looked forward to many more adventures to come.

The Magic of Springtime

Once upon a time in a small village nestled between rolling green hills, there lived a kind and sprightly old woman named Emma. Emma had lived a long and happy life, but as she grew older, she found herself feeling a bit more forgetful and less energetic than she used to be.

One bright spring morning, as Emma sat on her porch sipping her tea, she noticed that the world around her seemed to be coming alive. The trees were budding with vibrant green leaves, and colorful flowers were blooming everywhere. She closed her eyes and breathed in deeply, savoring the sweet fragrance of the fresh blooms.

As she sat there, she felt a strange sensation wash over her. Suddenly, she was no longer sitting on her porch but was transported to a lush garden filled with every flower imaginable. Emma felt a sense of wonder and joy as she wandered through the garden, taking in the vibrant colors and delightful fragrances.

As she walked, she noticed that each flower seemed to have a unique personality and story. The daffodils were full of energy and always seemed to be dancing in the breeze. The roses were proud and elegant, while the violets were shy and demure.

As Emma continued her stroll, she encountered a group of playful butterflies fluttering about. They invited her to join in their game of tag, and Emma couldn't help but laugh as they flitted about her, tickling her nose.

Eventually, Emma made her way to a cozy little cottage nestled among the flowers. Inside, she found a group of kind-hearted elves who welcomed her with open arms. They served her delicious tea and told her tales of their adventures in the garden.

Emma spent the entire day exploring the magical garden and learning from the whimsical creatures that lived there. As the sun began to set, she felt a sense of contentment and joy that she hadn't felt in years.

As she sat on her porch once again, watching the last rays of sunlight fade away, Emma realized that the magic of springtime had rekindled her imagination and renewed her zest for life. She knew that no matter how old she got, there would always be new adventures to discover and stories to tell.

And so, Emma spent the rest of her days sharing the tales of her magical garden with anyone who would listen. She knew that the memories she had made there would stay with her forever, and she was grateful for the gift of the magic of springtime.

The Sweet Taste of Memories

In a quaint little town nestled among the rolling green hills, there lived a charming old woman named Agatha. She was well-known in the town for her delicious homemade pies, which she would often bring to potlucks and community gatherings.

Agatha had always been proud of her baking skills, and she had passed down her recipes to her granddaughter, Lily. But as she grew older, Agatha found herself forgetting some of the finer details of her recipes, and her pies just didn't taste the same as they used to.

One day, while sitting on her porch and gazing out at the lush green hills, Agatha had a sudden inspiration. She decided to take a trip down memory lane by revisiting some of the places where she had collected the ingredients for her famous pies.

With a twinkle in her eye and a spring in her step, Agatha set off on her adventure. Her first stop was the local orchard, where she had picked apples for her pies for many years. As she walked among the trees, she could smell the crisp fragrance of the apples and hear the sound of leaves rustling in the breeze. She closed her eyes and savored the memories of happy times spent with her family and friends.

Next, she visited the farmer's market, where she had always bought the freshest ingredients for her pies. The bustling market was filled with colorful stalls selling fruits, vegetables, and baked goods. As Agatha strolled through the aisles, she could taste the sweetness of the fresh strawberries and smell the earthy aroma of the carrots.

As she continued on her journey, she visited a local bakery where she had once worked as a young woman. The smell of freshly baked bread and the sound of the whirring mixers brought back a flood of memories. She could remember the joy she felt when she had first discovered her love for baking.

Finally, Agatha returned home, her heart and mind filled with the sights, sounds, and smells of her memories. With renewed inspiration, she set to work on her pie recipes once again, this time with a new sense of joy and creativity.

As she baked her pies, she shared her memories with her granddaughter, Lily, who listened intently and laughed at the funny stories Agatha told.

Together, they experimented with new flavor combinations, and before long, they had created a masterpiece - a pie that captured the sweet taste of memories.

Agatha felt a sense of pride and accomplishment as she tasted the finished product. Her memory had been stimulated, her imagination had been reignited, and her sense of well-being had been elevated. And best of all, she had shared this journey with her granddaughter, passing down the traditions and memories of her family for generations to come.

The Surprise Visitor

Mrs. Emily Brown sat in her armchair, staring out the window. It was a beautiful day outside, the sun was shining, and a light breeze was blowing through the trees. But Emily felt lonely and bored. She missed her husband, who had passed away many years ago, and her children lived far away. She wished she had someone to talk to, someone to share her memories with.

Suddenly, she heard a knock at the door. She wondered who it could be since she wasn't expecting any visitors. She slowly got up and opened the door to find a young man standing on her doorstep.

"Good afternoon, ma'am," the young man said. "My name is Tom, and I'm here to deliver a surprise to you."

Emily was puzzled. She didn't know anyone named Tom, and she didn't expect any surprises. "I'm sorry, young man, but I think you have the wrong address," she said.

Tom smiled. "No, ma'am, I'm sure I'm in the

right place. You see, your granddaughter contacted me and asked me to deliver this to you." He handed her a small package wrapped in colorful paper.

Emily was intrigued. She didn't have any grandchildren, but she decided to open the package anyway. Inside, she found a beautiful photo album filled with pictures of her childhood, her wedding, and her family.

As she flipped through the pages, memories flooded her mind. She remembered the smell of her mother's cooking, the feel of her husband's hand in hers, the sound of her children's laughter. She laughed and cried as she relived those moments, and Tom sat patiently beside her, listening to her stories.

After a while, Emily realized that Tom was not just a delivery boy but a young man who cared about her. She invited him to stay for tea, and they talked for hours about their lives, their hopes, and their dreams. Emily felt grateful to have met Tom, and she knew that he had brought more than just a photo album into her life. He had brought companionship and joy.

As Tom left, Emily hugged him and whispered, "Thank you for being my surprise visitor today.

You have made my day, my week, and my year." Tom smiled and walked away, feeling happy to have made a difference in someone's life.

Emily sat back down in her armchair, feeling content and fulfilled. She realized that even in old age, life can be full of surprises and that there is always something to be grateful for. She looked at the photo album and whispered to herself, "I am not alone, and I am loved." And with that, she closed her eyes, feeling at peace.

The Sweetest Sound

Mrs. Agnes Wilson was an elderly woman who lived alone in her small cottage by the lake. She had lived there for over fifty years and had grown accustomed to the peaceful life in the countryside. She enjoyed spending her days tending to her garden, reading books, and watching the birds.

One day, while sitting on her porch, she heard a sound she hadn't heard in years. It was the sound of children's laughter. She looked out and saw a group of children playing in the meadow near her house. They were laughing, running, and having a great time. Agnes smiled and felt a pang of nostalgia. She remembered her own childhood, the fun she had, and the friends she made.

As she watched the children play, she noticed a young boy who seemed different from the others. He was standing by himself, looking sad and lost. Agnes felt sorry for him and decided to approach him.

"Hello, young man," she said. "What's wrong?"

The boy looked up at her and said, "I lost my

ball, and my friends won't play with me anymore."

Agnes smiled and said, "Don't worry. I'll help you find your ball."

Together they searched the meadow, and after a few minutes, they found the ball stuck in a tree. The boy was thrilled, and he hugged Agnes, thanking her for her help. He asked her if she wanted to play with him and his friends, and Agnes hesitated for a moment. She had forgotten how to play, and she didn't want to embarrass herself.

But then she remembered the joy she felt as a child, and she decided to join in. They played tag, hide and seek, and other games. Agnes laughed and ran with the children, feeling young again.

As the sun started to set, the children said goodbye and ran back to their homes. Agnes watched them go, feeling happy and grateful for the experience. She realized that she had missed out on so much in life by isolating herself, and she vowed to be more open to new experiences.

The next day, Agnes woke up to the sweetest sound she had ever heard: the sound of children's laughter. She smiled and knew that she had found a new purpose in life. She decided to start a children's club in her community, where children could come and play, learn, and have fun. She called it the "Sweetest Sound Club."

The club became very popular, and soon, Agnes had many young friends. She taught them about nature, gardening, and cooking. She shared her stories with them, and they shared theirs with her. She felt fulfilled and happy, knowing that she was making a difference in their lives.

Years went by, and Agnes grew old, but she never forgot the sweetest sound she had ever heard. It was the sound of children's laughter, and it had given her a new lease on life. She closed her eyes, feeling content, and whispered to herself, "Life is a playground, and I'm never too old to play."

The Great Pie Baking Competition

Agnes had always been known in her small town for her incredible baking skills. Her pies were the talk of the town, and everyone always looked forward to church and community events where Agnes would bring one of her famous pies.

As Agnes aged, she found herself feeling more and more isolated. Her friends had moved away or passed on, and she felt like she had lost her sense of purpose. That is until she heard about the town's annual pie baking competition.

Agnes had never entered the competition before, but she felt a surge of excitement as she decided to give it a try. She spent weeks perfecting her recipe and trying out new flavors and techniques.

The day of the competition arrived, and Agnes made her way to the town square with her best pie in hand. She saw a crowd of people gathered around a stage, and she made her way over to see what was going on.

To her surprise, the judges of the competition were none other than the town's three most notorious troublemakers - a mischievous trio who always seemed to be up to no good.

But Agnes didn't let that intimidate her. She confidently presented her pie to the judges and waited for their verdict. The judges tasted her pie, and their faces lit up with delight. They declared Agnes the winner of the competition.

Agnes was overjoyed. She had never felt so proud and accomplished. And as she made her way back home with her prize, she realized that she had regained a sense of purpose and belonging. She knew that she could still make a difference in her community, and that her pies would continue to bring joy to people for years to come.

The Great Pie Baking Competition had not only stimulated Agnes's memory of her love for baking, but it had also rekindled her sense of purpose and belonging. It had shown her that it's never too late to try something new and that you're never too old to make a difference.

The Bicycle Ride

Mr. Jones had always been a bit of a daredevil in his younger days, but at the ripe old age of 85, he had settled into a comfortable routine of sitting on his porch and watching the world go by. That is until he met his new neighbor, a spunky 7-year-old girl named Lily.

Lily had just gotten a new bicycle, and she loved to ride it up and down the street. One day, as she rode by Mr. Jones' house, she saw him sitting on the porch and stopped to say hello. Mr. Jones was taken aback by the bright-eyed little girl, but he couldn't help but smile at her enthusiasm.

Lily asked Mr. Jones if he wanted to take a ride on her bicycle, and he laughed at the idea. But something about the girl's persistence made him agree, and before he knew it, he was sitting on the back of her tiny bicycle, pedaling down the street.

As they rode, Mr. Jones felt the wind in his hair and the sun on his face. He smelled the freshly cut grass and heard the birds chirping in the trees. It was as if he was young again, and he couldn't help but laugh with joy.

Lily took him on a tour of the neighborhood, pointing out her favorite spots and telling him stories about her adventures. Mr. Jones felt his memory being stimulated as he thought back to his own childhood and the fun he used to have.

When they arrived back at Mr. Jones' house, he thanked Lily for the wonderful ride and gave her a big hug. As he watched her ride away, he realized that he had found a new sense of purpose and adventure in his life.

From that day on, Mr. Jones and Lily became the best of friends. They would take bicycle rides together every week, exploring new parts of the town and creating new memories. Mr. Jones felt his mind becoming more active, and his sense of well-being elevated. And it was all thanks to a little girl and her bicycle.

The Sweetest Fruit of Life

On a bright and sunny day, Mr. George, a man of ninety-one, sat on a park bench in the middle of the city, surrounded by the hustle and bustle of daily life. He had been a resident of the city his whole life, and had seen it change and grow, just as he had grown old. His mind was sharp, and his memories were vivid, but there was something he felt was missing in his life.

As he sat there, he noticed a young girl, no more than five years old, running around the park with her mother. The girl was full of energy and joy, and Mr. George couldn't help but smile at her infectious spirit. He thought back to his own childhood, and how he used to run around the park with his friends, playing games and enjoying the simple pleasures of life.

As he sat there lost in thought, he suddenly felt a tap on his shoulder. He turned around to see a young man, no more than thirty years old, standing behind him. The man introduced himself as Tom, and asked if he could sit and talk with him for a while.

Mr. George was hesitant at first, but something about the young man's friendly demeanor put him at ease. Tom sat down next to him, and they began to chat. They talked about the weather, and the city, and eventually they got onto the topic of life itself.

Tom asked Mr. George about his life, and he began to tell him stories of his youth, and the adventures he had. He spoke of the time he had climbed to the top of the tallest building in the city, and how he had felt on top of the world. He spoke of the time he had fallen in love, and how it had changed his life forever.

As he spoke, Mr. George began to feel a sense of joy and happiness that he hadn't felt in a long time. Tom listened intently to his stories, and soon they were laughing and joking like old friends.

As the day wore on, Mr. George began to realize that life was not about the big things, but about the small moments of joy and happiness that we experience every day. He realized that the sweetest fruit of life was not success or wealth, but the people we meet along the way, and the memories we create with them.

As the sun began to set, Tom stood up to leave, but not before giving Mr. George a warm embrace.

He thanked him for sharing his stories, and for reminding him of the beauty of life. Mr. George sat there for a few more moments, watching the young girl play with her mother, and feeling grateful for the simple pleasures of life.

As he got up to leave, he felt a sense of rejuvenation and a renewed appreciation for life. He knew that he would always cherish the memories he had created that day, and that he would always hold onto the sweetest fruit of life, the people we meet and the memories we create with them.

The Magic of Music

It was a hot summer day in the small town of Greenfield, where the sun was shining so bright that it felt like it could melt your skin off. The town was quiet, and there wasn't much happening on the streets. But in the park, a group of children were playing and laughing, running around and having the time of their lives. Among them was a little girl named Sarah, who was playing the violin.

Sarah was a shy and timid girl, but when she picked up her violin, she transformed into a different person. Her eyes would light up, and she would play with such passion and energy that it would fill the park with the most beautiful melodies. People passing by would stop to listen, and their hearts would fill with joy and happiness.

One day, while Sarah was playing her violin, an old man named George stopped to listen. He was a retired musician who had lost his hearing many years ago, and he had forgotten how beautiful music could be. But as he listened to Sarah's playing, he felt something inside of him stir. Memories of his youth came flooding back, and he was transported back to a time when music was everything to him.

George approached Sarah after she finished playing, and he told her how much he enjoyed her music. He asked her if she would be willing to teach him how to play the violin. Sarah was thrilled at the idea and agreed to teach him.

And so, Sarah and George began their journey together. Every day, they would meet in the park, and Sarah would teach George how to play the violin. At first, it was difficult for George, as he had to learn how to read music all over again. But Sarah was patient, and she encouraged him every step of the way.

As the weeks went by, George's playing improved, and he began to remember the joy he once felt when playing music. He started to feel young again, and he would spend hours practicing every day.

One day, Sarah surprised George by inviting him to play with her in the park. They played a duet, and the music they made together was so beautiful that it brought tears to the eyes of everyone who heard it.

From that day on, George and Sarah played

together every day in the park. People would stop to listen, and they would smile and tap their feet to the music. The park had become a place of joy and happiness, where people could forget about their troubles and lose themselves in the magic of music.

Years went by, and Sarah grew up and moved away. But George continued to play his violin every day in the park. He had rediscovered the joy of music, and he knew that it was something that he would never forget.

And so, the park remained a place of joy and happiness, where people could come to listen to George play his violin and remember the beauty of music. For George, it was a reminder that no matter how old you get, you can always find joy and happiness in the things you love.

The Beauty of Friendship

In the bustling city of New York, there lived two elderly friends, Lillian and Evelyn. They had been friends since childhood and had grown up together in the same neighborhood. They had shared many adventures and memories together over the years, and their friendship had only grown stronger with time.

One summer day, Lillian received a letter from her family who lived across the country, inviting her to come and visit them. Lillian was overjoyed at the invitation, but she didn't want to leave Evelyn alone. Evelyn had recently lost her husband, and Lillian didn't want her friend to be lonely while she was away.

So, Lillian came up with a plan. She arranged for a home health aide to visit Evelyn every day and keep her company. She also planned a surprise for Evelyn every day, leaving her small gifts and notes to remind her how much she loved her.

The first day, Evelyn woke up to find a basket of fresh fruit and a note from Lillian, telling her how much she meant to her. The second day, there was a bouquet of flowers waiting for her on the table. The third day, there was a homemade pie, still warm from the oven.

Evelyn was touched by her friend's thoughtfulness, and she started to look forward to the surprises every day. She also enjoyed spending time with the home health aide, who was kind and caring and always had a smile on her face.

As the days went by, Lillian sent Evelyn more gifts and notes, and she called her every day to check on her. Evelyn felt loved and cared for, and she knew that she had a true friend in Lillian.

When Lillian returned from her trip, she was happy to see Evelyn looking so well. She hugged her tightly and told her about all the adventures she had had with her family. Evelyn listened eagerly, and they laughed and reminisced about old times.

After that day, Lillian and Evelyn made a promise to each other that they would never let anything come between them. They knew that their friendship was rare and precious, and they would do anything to keep it alive.

And so, Lillian and Evelyn continued to spend their days together, enjoying each other's company and sharing the simple joys of life. They knew that life was short, but with each other by their side, they felt that they could conquer anything.

Their friendship was a reminder that no matter how old you get, you can still make new memories and find joy in the small things. It was a reminder that true friendship is a gift that should be cherished and nurtured, for it is one of the most beautiful things in life.

The Vibrant Tapestry of Life

As the sun rose over the sleepy town of Millfield, the colorful world came to life. The chirping of birds, the rustling of leaves, and the gentle breeze that carried the scent of flowers were all part of the daily routine. Amongst this colorful world, lived a young woman named Lily, whose heart was as bright as the sun itself.

Lily had a passion for adventure and would often spend her days exploring the town and discovering new sights and sounds. One day, she stumbled upon an old abandoned bookstore that had been shut down for years. But Lily was not deterred, she saw something special in that old bookstore and knew she had to save it.

She began working tirelessly to restore the old bookstore, cleaning the dust and cobwebs and bringing back the old books to life. As she worked, she discovered a dusty old book that caught her attention. It was a travel guidebook, full of colorful illustrations and detailed descriptions of exotic places around the world.

Lily couldn't resist the temptation and decided to

embark on a journey of her own, exploring the world one adventure at a time. She packed her bags, put on her walking shoes, and set out on her journey with the travel guidebook in hand.

Her first stop was a small village nestled in the rolling hills of Italy. The village was bursting with colors, from the bright reds of the ripe tomatoes to the deep greens of the lush vineyards. The air was filled with the aroma of fresh bread and the sounds of laughter and chatter.

As she wandered through the village, Lily stumbled upon a small café. She stepped inside, and her senses were overwhelmed by the aroma of freshly brewed coffee and the sight of colorful macarons on display. The café owner, a kind old woman named Maria, greeted her warmly and invited her to join in their conversation. They chatted for hours, sharing stories of their lives and adventures.

Lily's journey continued, and she traveled to many exotic places, from the bustling streets of Tokyo to the serene beaches of Bali. Everywhere she went, she made new friends and created unforgettable memories.

Years later, Lily returned home to Millfield, her

heart filled with love and her mind bursting with colorful memories. She reopened the old bookstore and filled it with her travel memoirs, inspiring others to embark on their own journeys and discover the beauty of the world.

As Lily sat in the bookstore, surrounded by the vibrant colors of her memories, she realized that life is a colorful journey, and every moment is an adventure waiting to be discovered.

The Sweet Aroma of Life

On a warm summer day, in a small town nestled in the heart of the countryside, lived a young woman named Emily. She had long golden hair that shimmered in the sun and a smile that lit up the room. Emily was known throughout the town for her sweet nature and kind heart.

One day, Emily received an unexpected gift - a basket of fresh, juicy strawberries from her neighbor's farm. As she held the basket, the sweet aroma of the strawberries filled her senses, taking her back to the days of her childhood.

She remembered how her grandmother would make homemade strawberry jam every summer, filling the house with the sweet aroma of strawberries. It was a time of joy and happiness, of family gatherings and endless laughter.

Emily decided to make her own strawberry jam, using the strawberries from her neighbor's farm. She spent hours in the kitchen, chopping and stirring, filling the house with the sweet aroma of strawberries.

As she worked, she thought about the sweet aroma of life. How it fills our senses with memories and emotions, transporting us back to the happy times of our past. She realized that life is like a basket of strawberries, sweet and full of flavor, waiting to be savored and enjoyed.

Emily's strawberry jam was a hit, and she began selling jars of it at the local farmer's market. People from all over the town came to taste her delicious jam, and Emily became known as the Strawberry Queen.

As the years went by, Emily's life was filled with joy and happiness. She married the love of her life and had children of her own. But the sweet aroma of strawberries remained a constant reminder of the simple joys of life.

Now, in her old age, Emily sits on her porch, watching the world go by. The sweet aroma of strawberries still fills her senses, and she smiles as she remembers the happy times of her past. She realizes that life is a tapestry of colors, sights, sounds, tastes, smells, and feelings, woven together to create a beautiful and vibrant masterpiece.

As the sun sets over the town, Emily takes a deep breath, filling her lungs with the sweet aroma of life.

She knows that life is a gift, a basket of strawberries waiting to be savored and enjoyed. And she is grateful for every sweet moment of it.

The Treasure Hunt

The sun shone brightly over the small town of Maplewood, as young Emily and her friends set out on their grand adventure. They were on a treasure hunt, a quest for the hidden riches of the mysterious Mr. Miller.

Emily was a bright and curious girl, with a heart full of wonder and a mind full of dreams. She was joined by her two best friends, Jack and Sarah, who were just as eager and excited as she was. They had heard rumors of Mr. Miller's treasure, and they were determined to find it.

Their journey took them through the winding streets of the town, past colorful houses and shops, and into the quiet woods beyond. They climbed over fallen logs, waded through streams, and ducked under low-hanging branches, following a map that Emily had carefully drawn.

As they traveled, they talked and laughed and imagined all the wonderful things they might find. They dreamed of gold and jewels and magical objects that could grant their wildest wishes.

But as they drew closer to their goal, they began to realize that the true treasure wasn't the material wealth they had imagined. It was the journey itself, the thrill of the chase, the joy of discovery, and the bonds of friendship that had grown stronger with each step they took.

Finally, they came to a small clearing in the woods, where they found a weathered old chest. With trembling hands, they lifted the lid, and their hearts filled with wonder and amazement.

Inside the chest, there was no gold or jewels, no magical objects. Instead, there was a note from Mr. Miller, explaining that the real treasure was the journey they had taken, and the memories they had made along the way.

Emily, Jack, and Sarah smiled at each other, feeling grateful and blessed to have each other, and to have experienced such a wonderful adventure. They knew that they would treasure this memory forever, and that it would always fill their hearts with joy and warmth.

As they made their way back home, they talked and laughed and shared their favorite moments of the journey. And though they had not found the material riches they had sought, they had found something much more valuable - a sense of wonder, a spirit of adventure, and a deep appreciation for the beauty and magic of the world around them.

A Garden of Memories

Mrs. Edna lived in a small cottage by the lake. She was a spry old lady, always up for an adventure. Her cottage was painted pink, and it had a lovely garden filled with flowers of all colors. Every morning, she would wake up early and tend to her garden, humming a tune as she watered the plants.

One day, as she was walking by the lake, she noticed a young boy sitting on the edge, looking gloomy. His name was Peter, and he had just moved to the town with his family. Mrs. Edna could sense that he was feeling lonely and homesick.

She sat down next to him and struck up a conversation. They talked about the lake, the trees, and the birds. Soon, Peter's face lit up, and he started to smile. Mrs. Edna invited him to her cottage, and they spent the day exploring her garden.

"Look at these roses," Mrs. Edna said, pointing to a bed of red flowers. "They smell so sweet, and they remind me of my first love."

Peter listened intently as she told him stories about her youth. He was fascinated by the colorful tales of adventure and love. As they walked around the garden, they noticed a butterfly fluttering nearby. It was a beautiful monarch butterfly with orange and black wings.

"Did you know that butterflies are a symbol of change and transformation?" Mrs. Edna said. "They remind us that life is always changing, and we must learn to adapt to new situations."

Peter nodded, and they continued their walk. They stopped by a patch of herbs, and Mrs. Edna picked some mint and basil leaves. "These herbs are not only delicious but also have healing properties," she said.

As they sat down for tea, Mrs. Edna brought out a tray of cookies that she had baked earlier that day. "These cookies are my secret recipe," she said, smiling mischievously.

Peter took a bite and exclaimed, "These are delicious! You should sell them in a bakery."

Mrs. Edna laughed and said, "I don't have the energy to run a bakery, but I'm glad you like them."

As the sun started to set, Peter got up to leave. Mrs. Edna hugged him and said, "You're always welcome here, Peter. And remember, life is like a garden. You have to nurture it, and it will bloom beautifully."

Peter walked away, feeling grateful and happy. Mrs. Edna sat down in her rocking chair, watching the sun disappear behind the horizon. She thought about her life, filled with colorful memories and adventures. She felt content and grateful for everything she had.

As she closed her eyes, she heard the faint sound of music, and she smiled. It was the same tune she had hummed that morning while tending to her garden. It was a reminder that life was beautiful, and every day was an adventure waiting to happen.

The Gift of Laughter

Mr. Bertie was a jolly old man with a twinkle in his eye and a quick wit. He lived in a small apartment in the heart of the city, surrounded by bustling crowds and towering buildings. Despite his humble surroundings, he was a man of great wealth - he possessed the gift of laughter.

Every day, he would sit on a park bench, watching the people go by. He would crack jokes and tell stories, making everyone around him laugh. His laughter was infectious, and soon, people started to gather around him, eager to hear his jokes and anecdotes.

One day, as he was sitting on the bench, he noticed a young woman walking by. She looked sad and forlorn, and Mr. Bertie could sense that she needed a good laugh.

He approached her and said, "Excuse me, miss. You look like you could use a good joke. What do you get when you cross a snowman and a shark?"

The woman looked puzzled and said, "I don't

know. What?"

"Frostbite!" Mr. Bertie exclaimed, bursting into laughter.

The woman couldn't help but laugh, and soon, she was chuckling and smiling. Mr. Bertie continued to tell her jokes and stories, and by the end of their conversation, the woman's spirits were lifted.

As she was about to leave, Mr. Bertie handed her a small card. "Keep this with you, my dear. It's a gift from me to you."

The woman opened the card and read the words written inside: "The gift of laughter is the greatest gift of all."

The woman smiled and said, "Thank you, Mr. Bertie. You've given me a wonderful gift today."

Mr. Bertie tipped his hat and said, "My pleasure, my dear. Remember, life is too short not to laugh."

As he watched the woman walk away, Mr. Bertie felt a sense of satisfaction. He knew that he had made a difference in her day, and that was all that mattered.

As the sun started to set, Mr. Bertie walked back to his apartment, humming a tune. He thought about his life, filled with laughter and joy, and he felt grateful for everything he had. He knew that his gift of laughter was something special, something that could bring happiness to even the saddest of hearts.

And as he lay down to sleep that night, he knew that tomorrow would be another day filled with laughter, joy, and the gift of life.

Rediscovering Joy: The Unforgettable Journey of Mr. Tompkins

Mr. Tompkins sat alone in his small apartment, surrounded by stacks of books and piles of papers. His weathered face bore the marks of age and experience, and his wrinkled hands trembled as he reached for his pen. He had spent his entire life as a historian, documenting the stories of those who had gone before him. But now, as he sat alone, he realized that he had neglected to document his own story.

As he sat there, lost in thought, a knock at the door interrupted his reverie. He rose slowly, shuffling towards the door. Upon opening it, he was greeted by a young woman with bright eyes and a warm smile.

"Hello, Mr. Tompkins," she said. "My name is Sarah, and I work at the local library. We're starting a new program for seniors, and we thought you might be interested in participating."

Mr. Tompkins was hesitant at first. He had spent so long in his own world that the thought of interacting with others seemed daunting. But something about Sarah's kindness drew him in, and he found himself nodding in agreement.

And so began Mr. Tompkins' journey, a journey that would take him to places he had never imagined. He met new people, each with their own unique story to tell. He visited places he had only read about in books, experiencing them firsthand with the help of his newfound friends. And he discovered a joy and vitality that he had long thought lost.

As the weeks went on, Mr. Tompkins' mind became clearer, and his spirit brighter. He reveled in the simple pleasures of life, savoring the taste of fresh fruit and the sound of children playing in the park. And as he shared his own story with those around him, he found that it was not only his memory that was stimulated, but his heart as well.

One day, as he sat with Sarah and the other seniors, Mr. Tompkins realized that he had found what he had been searching for his whole life. It wasn't the stories of others that had captivated him, but the stories that he himself had yet to live. And with that realization came a new sense of purpose, a new sense of adventure.

As he left the library that day, Mr. Tompkins

knew that his journey was far from over. But he was filled with a sense of hope and excitement, knowing that each step he took would be his own, and that each day would hold new wonders and new joys.

And so, with a spring in his step and a twinkle in his eye, Mr. Tompkins set out on the sweetest journey of all, the journey of life.

The Gift of Giving

Charlie was a young man who loved nothing more than making people smile. He was known throughout his small town for his kindness and generosity, and he made it his mission to bring joy to the lives of those around him.

One day, as he was walking through town, Charlie came across an old woman selling flowers on the street corner. The woman looked tired and sad, and Charlie could tell that she wasn't having much luck selling her wares.

Without a second thought, Charlie approached the woman and asked if he could buy all of her flowers. The woman was hesitant at first, but Charlie's infectious smile and warm demeanor soon won her over.

As he walked away with the armfuls of flowers, Charlie began to think of all the people he could give them to. He knew that the local hospital was filled with patients who could use a little cheer, and he decided that was where he would start.

And so Charlie spent the rest of the day

delivering flowers to the hospital, brightening the rooms of patients and bringing smiles to their faces. But he didn't stop there. He continued to give away flowers to anyone he saw who looked like they could use a pick-me-up.

As the day wore on, Charlie began to feel tired and hungry. But he didn't let that stop him. He knew that he had a mission, and he wasn't going to let anyone down.

Finally, as the sun began to set and the last of the flowers had been given away, Charlie collapsed onto a park bench, exhausted but elated. It had been a long and tiring day, but he knew that he had made a difference in the lives of so many people.

As he sat there catching his breath, a small boy approached him. The boy had been watching Charlie all day, and he was amazed by his kindness and generosity.

"Excuse me, mister," the boy said. "I don't have any money, but I want to give you something."

And with that, the boy handed Charlie a small, wilted flower that he had picked from a nearby garden.

Charlie felt tears well up in his eyes as he looked at the little flower. It may not have been much, but it was the most precious gift he had ever received. And in that moment, he realized that the true gift of giving was not in what you received, but in the joy that you brought to others.

As he walked home that night, Charlie felt a sense of purpose and fulfillment that he had never felt before. He knew that he would spend the rest of his life spreading kindness and generosity wherever he went, and that he would never forget the lesson that the little boy had taught him.

And so, with a heart full of love and a smile on his face, Charlie set out to make the world a better place, one small act of kindness at a time.

The Secret of the Old Watch

Mrs. Perkins was an elderly woman who lived alone in a small house at the edge of town. She had always been a bit of a recluse, rarely leaving her home except to go to the grocery store or church on Sundays.

One day, a young man named Jack was walking past Mrs. Perkins' house when he noticed that the front door was ajar. Concerned, he approached the house and knocked on the door. When there was no answer, he pushed the door open and stepped inside.

The house was dimly lit, and Jack could see that Mrs. Perkins' living room was cluttered with old furniture and stacks of newspapers. As he made his way through the room, he noticed an old watch lying on the coffee table.

The watch was rusted and tarnished, and it looked like it had been sitting there for years. But there was something about it that caught Jack's eye, and he picked it up to examine it more closely.

As he turned the watch over in his hands, he

noticed that the back was engraved with a name and a date. The name was that of a man named Harry, and the date was over twenty years ago.

Jack was curious about the watch and wondered what its story might be. He decided to ask Mrs. Perkins about it, but when he knocked on her bedroom door, there was no answer.

Feeling uneasy, Jack decided to leave the house and come back another time. But as he was leaving, he noticed a young woman walking up to the house.

The woman introduced herself as Mrs. Perkins' granddaughter, and Jack explained that he had stopped by to check on her grandmother. The granddaughter looked worried and told Jack that Mrs. Perkins had been in the hospital for the past week.

As they talked, Jack showed the granddaughter the old watch and asked her if she knew anything about it. The granddaughter's eyes widened as she recognized the watch.

"That belonged to my grandfather," she said. "He passed away over twenty years ago, and my grandmother has kept it with her ever since. She never talks about him, but I know that he meant a lot to her."

As they stood there on the porch, Jack realized that he had stumbled upon a secret that Mrs. Perkins had been keeping for years. He felt a pang of sadness for the old woman, who had been living with her memories and her grief for so long.

But he also felt a sense of hope. Perhaps now that the secret was out, Mrs. Perkins could begin to heal and move on with her life.

As he walked away from the house, Jack felt grateful for the small glimpse into Mrs. Perkins' life that the old watch had given him. He knew that he would never forget the sense of mystery and wonder that it had brought him, and he hoped that Mrs. Perkins would find peace knowing that her secret had finally been revealed.

The Gift of the Magi

It was Christmas Eve, and Sarah and John were a young couple living in a small apartment in the city. They loved each other deeply but had no money to buy each other gifts for the holiday.

As they sat together on the couch, Sarah sighed and said, "I wish I could give you something special for Christmas. I love you so much."

John looked at her and said, "I feel the same way. I wish I could give you something, too."

Suddenly, Sarah had an idea. "What if we each sold our most prized possession to buy a gift for the other?" she said.

John looked skeptical but then smiled. "That's a great idea," he said.

So they both set out to sell their most valuable possessions. Sarah had a beautiful set of long hair that she had been growing for years, and John had a pocket watch that had been passed down in his family for generations.

As they made their way through the city, they were both nervous and excited. They knew that the gifts they would give each other would be priceless, but they also felt a sense of sadness at parting with their cherished possessions.

Finally, they met up at a street corner, each holding a small package. They hugged each other tightly, then opened their gifts.

Sarah gasped when she saw what John had given her. It was a beautiful comb made of the finest materials, perfect for her long hair. John had sold his pocket watch to buy it.

John's heart swelled with love when he saw what Sarah had given him. She had bought him a chain for his pocket watch, knowing how much it meant to him. She had sold her hair to buy it.

Tears filled their eyes as they hugged each other, knowing that they had given each other the most precious gifts of all - the gift of their love and devotion.

As they sat together in their small apartment, holding hands and watching the snow fall outside their window, they knew that they would never forget this special Christmas Eve, the night they gave each other the greatest gift of all.

Sweet Friendship: A Tale of Chocolates and Memories

In the bustling streets of New York, there lived an old man named George. He had lived a long and fulfilling life, but as he grew older, he felt himself slipping away from the world he had always known. His memories were beginning to fade, and his body was slowing down. However, George was determined to stay active and keep his mind alive, no matter what.

One day, as George was walking down the street, he stumbled upon a candy shop. The shop had been there for as long as he could remember, but he had never been inside. Curious, George decided to take a look. As he walked in, the sweet scent of chocolate and sugar filled his nostrils, and he was transported back to his childhood.

Behind the counter stood a young woman with a bright smile. Her name was Emma, and she was the owner of the candy shop. As George browsed through the shelves, Emma struck up a conversation with him. They talked about their favorite candies, their memories of childhood, and their dreams for the future. It was a refreshing change of pace for George, who had grown accustomed to the loneliness of old age.

Over the next few weeks, George would stop by the candy shop every day to chat with Emma. They became fast friends, sharing stories and laughs over cups of hot chocolate and plates of candy. George felt like a young boy again, with his whole life ahead of him.

One day, as George was about to leave the candy shop, Emma handed him a small box. "I made these especially for you," she said with a smile. "I hope you like them."

George opened the box to find a selection of homemade chocolates, each one carefully crafted and wrapped in shiny foil. He took a bite of one and closed his eyes in pure bliss. It was the sweetest thing he had ever tasted.

As he savored the chocolates, George realized that he had been given the greatest gift of all - the gift of friendship. Emma had reminded him that there was still joy and love to be found in the world, no matter how old he was.

From that day on, George continued to visit the candy shop, not just for the sweet treats but for the sweet company of his new friend. He learned that it's never too late to make new memories and create new friendships, and that life can still be full of surprises, even in old age.

As George walked home with a smile on his face, he felt a sense of peace and contentment that he hadn't felt in years. He knew that he had been given a second chance at life, and he wasn't going to waste it.

And so, the old man and the young woman continued to share their love of candy and their love of life, proving that age is just a number, and that friendship knows no bounds.

The Metronome of Life: A Musical Legacy

In a small town nestled in the countryside, there lived an old man named Harold. He had lived in the same house his entire life and had seen the town change around him. As he grew older, Harold found solace in his love for music. He had been playing the piano since he was a young boy, and it was the one thing that had remained constant in his life.

One day, as Harold was playing his piano, he heard a knock on the door. It was a young girl named Lily, who lived next door. She had always been fascinated by Harold's piano playing and had been listening to him through the wall.

"Can I listen to you play?" she asked with a smile.

Harold welcomed her into his home and played a few tunes for her. Lily was mesmerized by his music and begged him to teach her how to play.

Over the next few weeks, Harold taught Lily how to play the piano. He shared his love of music with her, and together they played duets and sang songs.

Lily was a natural, and Harold was proud to have passed on his love of music to the next generation.

As the months went by, Harold's health began to decline. He found it harder and harder to play the piano, and he knew that his time was running out. One day, he called Lily over to his house and handed her a small box.

"I want you to have this," he said with a smile. "It's my old metronome. I used it when I was your age and learning to play the piano. I want you to use it to keep time and keep your music on track."

Lily took the metronome and thanked Harold for the gift. She knew how much it meant to him to pass on his love of music, and she was honored to continue his legacy.

Years went by, and Harold passed away. But his love of music lived on through Lily. She continued to play the piano and became a renowned musician in her own right. She never forgot the gift that Harold had given her and always kept his metronome on her piano.

As Lily sat down to play, she set the metronome ticking, and it was as if Harold was right there beside her, guiding her music and filling her heart with joy. She knew that Harold's gift had been more than just a metronome - it was a reminder that music had the power to connect people, no matter how old or young, and that it could bring joy and comfort to anyone who was willing to listen.

And so, the gift of music was passed down from generation to generation, a legacy that Harold had started and Lily had continued, proving that sometimes the greatest gifts are the ones that keep on giving.

The Painting of Memories

Mrs. Lorraine was a kind and gentle soul who had lived in the same house for more than sixty years. Her house was filled with mementos and keepsakes, each one holding a special memory that she cherished. But there was one thing in her house that was her most prized possession - a painting of her late husband.

The painting had been done by a local artist named Sarah, who had been a dear friend of Mrs. Lorraine's for many years. Sarah had captured the essence of Mrs. Lorraine's husband perfectly, and the painting was a constant reminder of the love they had shared.

As the years went by, Mrs. Lorraine grew older, and her health began to decline. She knew that she would soon have to leave her beloved home and move to a retirement community. But there was one thing she couldn't bear to leave behind - the painting of her husband.

One day, she called Sarah over to her house and asked her a favor. "I want you to take the painting with you," she said. "I don't want it to be left behind when I'm gone."

Sarah was touched by Mrs. Lorraine's request and agreed to take the painting with her. She hung it in her own living room, where it became a conversation piece for all her visitors. Everyone who saw the painting commented on how beautiful it was and how much it captured the love between Mrs. Lorraine and her husband.

Years went by, and Sarah grew old herself. She knew that it was time to pass on the painting to someone else, but she didn't know who. Then, one day, she received a call from a woman named Emily. Emily had been Mrs. Lorraine's neighbor for many years and had always admired the painting.

"I heard that you have the painting of Mrs. Lorraine's husband," Emily said. "I was wondering if you would be willing to sell it to me."

Sarah knew that she could never sell the painting - it was too precious and held too many memories. But she also knew that Mrs. Lorraine would have wanted it to go to someone who appreciated it as much as she did.

And so, Sarah gifted the painting to Emily, who hung it in her own home. Every time Emily looked at the painting, she felt a connection to Mrs. Lorraine and her late husband. It was as if the painting held a piece of their love, which she could feel in her heart.

Years went by, and Emily grew old herself. She knew that it was time to pass on the painting to someone else, but she didn't know who. Then, one day, she received a call from a young couple who had just bought the house next door.

"We saw the painting through the window," the woman said. "We were wondering if you could tell us more about it."

Emily smiled and told them the story of Mrs. Lorraine, her husband, and the painting that had brought them all together. She knew that the painting would continue to hold a special place in people's hearts for many years to come, just as it had for her and for Mrs. Lorraine.

And so, the painting of memories continued to pass from person to person, connecting them all in a web of love and nostalgia, reminding them that the most precious possessions are the ones that hold the memories of the people we have loved and lost.

Adventures in Aging: Mr. Franklin's Colorful Memories

Mr. Franklin was a man who had lived a long and colorful life. He had traveled far and wide, met countless people, and seen countless places. His eyes had beheld the beauty of the world, and his ears had heard the sweet sounds of music and laughter.

Now, in his old age, Mr. Franklin loved nothing more than to sit in his favorite armchair and reflect on his past adventures. He would close his eyes and let his mind wander back in time, savoring the memories of his travels.

One day, as Mr. Franklin was enjoying his afternoon tea, a knock came at the door. He shuffled over to answer it and found a young woman standing there.

"Good afternoon, sir," she said politely. "My name is Lucy, and I work at the local nursing home. We are looking for volunteers to come and spend time with our residents, and I was wondering if you would be interested?"

Mr. Franklin was intrigued. He had never thought of himself as a volunteer before, but the idea of spending time with other people his age appealed to him. So, he agreed to visit the nursing home the following day.

When Mr. Franklin arrived at the nursing home, he was greeted by a group of elderly residents who were sitting in the communal area. They looked up as he approached, and one woman called out, "Hello there! Come and join us!"

Mr. Franklin smiled and sat down next to her. She introduced herself as Mrs. Jenkins and asked him about his life.

"I've had quite the adventure, Mrs. Jenkins," Mr. Franklin said with a chuckle. "I've traveled all over the world and met all kinds of people. I've seen mountains and oceans and deserts. I've tasted exotic foods and heard beautiful music."

The other residents listened intently as Mr. Franklin regaled them with stories of his adventures. He described the colorful markets of Morocco, the ancient temples of Japan, and the bustling streets of New York City.

As he spoke, Mr. Franklin felt a warmth in his

heart. It was wonderful to share his memories with others and to feel their enthusiasm for his stories. He had forgotten how much joy he could bring to people just by sharing his experiences.

The afternoon flew by, and before he knew it, it was time to go home. As he left the nursing home, Mr. Franklin felt a sense of contentment that he hadn't felt in a long time. He realized that even though he was getting older, he still had so much to give to the world.

From that day on, Mr. Franklin visited the nursing home regularly. He shared his stories with the other residents and listened to theirs in return. He made new friends and found that he had a sense of purpose that he had been missing.

And as he sat in his armchair each evening, reflecting on his day, Mr. Franklin realized that his adventures were far from over. He was still traveling, still meeting new people, and still seeing the beauty of the world. And he knew that as long as he kept sharing his experiences with others, he would never truly grow old.

"So, Mrs. Jenkins," Mr. Franklin said with a twinkle in his eye. "Where would you like me to take you on our next adventure?"

The Last Dance

Mrs. Brown had been living in the same house for over 50 years. She had raised her children there, welcomed her grandchildren, and spent countless hours tending to her beautiful garden. But now, as she sat in her armchair staring out the window, she knew that it was time to say goodbye to the place that had been her home for so long.

Her children had all grown up and moved away, and her husband had passed away a few years ago. Mrs. Brown knew that she could no longer manage the house on her own, and that it was time to move into a retirement community.

On the day of her move, Mrs. Brown sat in her empty living room, surrounded by boxes and memories. She felt a sense of sadness and loss, but also a sense of gratitude for all the years she had spent in the house.

As she was packing up her things, she came across an old record player and a stack of records. She had not played them in years, but she knew that she had to listen to them one last time before she left.

Mrs. Brown put on one of her favorite records and sat down in the middle of the empty living room. As the music filled the space, she closed her eyes and let herself be transported back in time.

She remembered the parties she used to host, with friends and family dancing in the living room. She remembered her husband twirling her around the room, their laughter ringing out over the music. She remembered the warmth and joy that had filled the house during those moments.

Mrs. Brown opened her eyes and looked around the empty room. She knew that this was the last dance in this house, the final goodbye to a place that had held so many memories.

But as the music continued to play, she realized that the memories would live on. They would live on in the hearts of her family and friends, and in the stories they would tell about the house and the moments they had shared there.

And with that realization, Mrs. Brown felt a sense of peace. She knew that it was time to move on to the next chapter of her life, but that the memories of the past would always be with her, like a warm embrace that would never let her go.

The Lemonade Stand

It was a scorching hot summer day in the small town of Millfield, where the sun was beating down on the dusty sidewalks and the grass was wilting under the heat. The air was filled with the sound of crickets and the scent of freshly cut grass.

At the corner of the street, a little girl named Lily had set up a lemonade stand with her older neighbor, Mr. Green. Mr. Green was a kind old man who had lived in Millfield for as long as anyone could remember. His smile was warm and his voice was gentle, and he had a twinkle in his eye that made Lily feel safe and happy.

Together, they had made a big pitcher of lemonade, and it was the most delicious drink Lily had ever tasted. The lemons were tangy, the sugar was sweet, and the ice cubes were cold and refreshing.

As they poured the lemonade into cups and handed them to the passersby, Lily chatted with Mr. Green and listened to his stories. He told her about the old days when Millfield was just a little village with dirt roads and gas lamps, and the people were as friendly as they were poor.

He told her about the time he met his wife, Mary, at the town fair, and how they fell in love over a plate of funnel cake. He told her about the time he saw a circus come to town and watched the elephants parade down Main Street.

Lily loved listening to Mr. Green's stories, and she loved how the lemonade stand brought people together. Some customers were young kids like her, with sticky fingers and big grins. Others were older folks, with wrinkles and walking sticks and fond memories of their own.

One customer in particular caught Lily's attention. It was an old man with a white beard and a twinkle in his eye, just like Mr. Green. He wore a faded blue shirt and a cap with a fish on it, and he carried a fishing rod over his shoulder.

"Hey there, young lady," he said to Lily. "That's a mighty fine lemonade stand you've got there."

"Thank you, sir," Lily said, smiling up at him. "Would you like a cup of lemonade?"

"I sure would," he said, and took a sip. "Mmm, that's good stuff. You know, I used to fish in the creek just down the road when I was your age. Caught myself some big ones, too."

"Really?" Lily said, her eyes widening. "That sounds amazing."

"It was," the old man said, nodding. "But I'll tell you what's even more amazing. You're making memories right now, young lady. Memories that you'll cherish for a long time to come."

Lily looked at Mr. Green, who was nodding and smiling. She looked at the customers, who were laughing and chatting. She looked at the lemonade, which was still cold and refreshing. And she realized that the old man was right.

She was making memories.

As the sun began to set and the shadows grew long, Lily and Mr. Green closed up the lemonade stand and counted their earnings. It wasn't much, but it was enough to buy some more lemons and sugar for next time.

As they walked home, Lily thought about the old man's words. She thought about the memories she had made that day, and the memories she would make in the future. She thought about Mr. Green and his stories, and about the people who had stopped by the lemonade stand.

And she realized that the lemonade stand wasn't just about selling lemonade. It was about making memories, and about bringing people together.

It was about the sense of community that could be created with something as simple as a cup of lemonade.

As Lily and Mr. Green walked, they passed by the old man with the fishing rod again. He smiled at them and tipped his cap.

"Good luck with the lemonade stand, young lady," he said. "And don't forget what I told you. You're making memories."

Lily smiled back at him and felt a warm sense of happiness in her chest. She knew that she would always remember this day, and that the lemonade stand would always hold a special place in her heart.

Years later, when Lily was all grown up and had children of her own, she would often think back to that hot summer day in Millfield. She would remember the taste of the lemonade, the sound of Mr. Green's voice, and the feeling of community that had been created at the lemonade stand.

And she would smile, knowing that the memories she had made that day would stay with her forever.

.

The Magician's Assistant

Old Mrs. Withers lived alone in a small apartment above the magic shop where she had worked as an assistant for many years. She had always loved magic, with its intricate illusions and hidden secrets. But now, in her old age, she was often lonely and longed for the days when she had been part of the magic show.

One day, a young magician named Max walked into the shop. He had just moved to town and was looking for a new assistant. Mrs. Withers was hesitant at first, but Max was charming and eager to learn from her.

Over the weeks and months that followed, Max and Mrs. Withers rehearsed their act tirelessly, perfecting each trick and making sure that everything was just right. Max was a quick learner, and soon he was performing for small audiences at the local coffee shop.

Mrs. Withers watched from the sidelines, proud of the young man she had taught. But as Max's fame grew, she began to feel left behind. She was no longer needed for the shows, and Max was often too busy to stop by and say hello.

One day, Mrs. Withers decided to visit Max at the coffee shop. She was surprised to find that he was performing a new trick - one that she had never seen before. Max had taken the old trick of sawing a woman in half and turned it into something truly spectacular.

The audience was amazed as Max placed Mrs. Withers into the box and began to saw it in half. But as the sawblade cut through the wood, something strange happened. Mrs. Withers disappeared!

The audience gasped, and Max looked around frantically for his assistant. Suddenly, there was a rustling noise from behind the curtain. Mrs. Withers emerged, grinning from ear to ear.

"You never stop learning in this business," she said to Max. "And I still have a few tricks up my sleeve."

Max hugged Mrs. Withers, realizing how much he had taken her for granted. He had been so focused on his own success that he had forgotten the woman who had taught him everything he knew.

From that day on, Max and Mrs. Withers performed together as a team. The audience loved their act, and they became known as the most dynamic duo in magic.

As they took their final bow each night, Mrs. Withers would look out at the crowd and feel a sense of pride and joy. She had found a new family in Max and the magic shop, and she knew that she would always be a part of the show.

The Candy Shop on Main Street

Once upon a time, on a bright sunny day, in the heart of a small town, nestled between two old brick buildings, there stood a quaint little candy shop. It was run by an old man named Mr. Jones, who had a smile for everyone that passed by.

One day, a young girl named Lily walked into the candy shop. She was curious about the shop because she had heard stories about it from her grandmother. The old lady had told her that the candy shop had been around for generations, and that Mr. Jones was the kindest man in town.

As Lily entered the shop, she was greeted by the sweet aroma of candy and the sound of laughter. The walls were covered in colorful jars of candy, and the shelves were stacked with every kind of treat imaginable.

Mr. Jones welcomed her with a warm smile, and asked her what kind of candy she liked. Lily told him that she loved everything, and Mr. Jones began to tell her the story of how he had started the candy shop many years ago.

He spoke of how he had always loved candy as a boy, and how he had saved up his pennies to buy his first jar of candy. He had enjoyed it so much that he had decided to start his own candy shop, so that he could share the joy with others.

As he spoke, Lily listened intently, and she couldn't help but be drawn in by the kindness and passion of Mr. Jones. She asked him how he had managed to keep the candy shop open for so long, and Mr. Jones replied that it was all thanks to the people of the town.

He told her that every day, people from all walks of life came into the shop, and that he had made many friends over the years. They would tell him stories about their lives, and he would listen with a sympathetic ear.

Suddenly, the door opened, and in walked a group of elderly ladies, who greeted Mr. Jones with hugs and kisses. They were regular customers of the candy shop, and they had come to buy their favorite candies.

As they chatted, Lily watched them with wonder. She saw how happy they were, and how they were always eager to share their stories with Mr. Jones. She realized that the candy shop wasn't just a place to buy candy, but a community of people who cared for each other.

Before she left, Lily bought a bag of her favorite candy and said goodbye to Mr. Jones. As she walked out of the shop, she felt a sense of happiness and contentment that she had never felt before. She knew that she would always remember the candy shop on Main Street, and the kindness of Mr. Jones.

As for Mr. Jones, he continued to run the candy shop for many more years, and it remained a beloved fixture of the town. And whenever someone asked him how he managed to keep the shop open for so long, he would simply smile and say, "It's all thanks to the people of the town."

The Last Leaf

Samantha was a young artist living in a small apartment in the city. She had moved there to pursue her passion for painting, but lately, she had lost her inspiration. Her paintings lacked the magic they once had, and she felt empty inside.

One autumn day, Samantha noticed that the tree outside her window was losing its leaves. Every day, she would watch as another leaf fell to the ground, until only one leaf remained.

She couldn't help but feel a connection to that last leaf. It was a symbol of her own struggles, her own fight to hold on to her creativity and passion.

One night, Samantha fell ill with a fever. Her friends gathered around her, hoping for her recovery, but the doctor was not optimistic. They all feared the worst.

As Samantha lay in her bed, she watched as the last leaf on the tree outside her window held on, despite the wind and rain. It was a small, brave thing, holding on until the very end.

Days passed, and Samantha's condition did not improve. Her friends grew more and more worried, and even the doctor had given up hope.

One day, her friend Sue came to visit her, and Samantha asked her to open the window so she could see the tree. To her surprise, the last leaf was still there, clinging to the branch.

Sue saw the look of hope in Samantha's eyes and said, "You know, I heard a story once about a young artist who was losing her inspiration. She watched as the last leaf on a tree outside her window held on, and it gave her the courage to keep going."

Samantha smiled weakly, feeling a renewed sense of hope. She knew that if that last leaf could hold on, she could too.

As the days passed, Samantha slowly began to recover. And one morning, when she looked out her window, she saw that the last leaf was still there, still holding on.

It was a small thing, but it gave her the strength to keep fighting, to keep creating, to keep living.

Years later, when Samantha had become a

successful artist, she returned to that small apartment in the city and visited the tree outside her window. The last leaf was long gone, but the memory of its bravery had stayed with her, a reminder of the power of hope and the strength of the human spirit.

"Unexpected Gifts: A Tale of Generosity and the True Meaning of Giving

Lena was a wealthy woman who had everything she could ever want. She lived in a large mansion, wore expensive clothes, and had all the latest gadgets. But despite all her possessions, she felt empty inside.

One day, Lena decided to volunteer at a local charity organization. She thought it would be a good way to give back to the community and maybe fill the void she felt inside.

At the charity, Lena met a young boy named Tommy. He was bright and curious, but he had nothing. He wore ragged clothes and had no toys or books to call his own. Lena felt a pang of sadness as she looked at him.

She decided to give him a gift, a brand new laptop. She thought it would be a nice gesture, something that would help him with his studies and maybe inspire him to reach for his dreams.

Tommy was thrilled with the gift and thanked Lena. She felt good, happy that she had made a difference in someone's life.

Days passed, and Lena went about her life, feeling good about her charitable act. But then, something unexpected happened.

Lena received a letter in the mail. It was from Tommy, and he had written her a thank you note. But it was not what Lena expected.

In the note, Tommy wrote that he was grateful for the laptop, but he realized that it was not the gift he truly needed. What he really needed was someone to talk to, someone to listen to him and help him navigate the challenges he faced in life.

Lena was shocked. She had never thought about it that way. She had thought that her gift was all Tommy needed, but he had shown her that the gift of giving was not just about material possessions.

She decided to visit Tommy at the charity organization and talk to him. They talked for hours, and Lena learned about Tommy's dreams and aspirations. She realized that he had so much potential, and she wanted to help him in any way she could.

Together, they came up with a plan. Lena would use her resources and connections to help Tommy get the education and support he needed to achieve his dreams.

In the end, Lena realized that the gift of giving was not just about material possessions. It was about giving of oneself, about listening and supporting others, and about making a difference in someone's life.

The Painter and the Garden

It was a warm summer day, and the sun was shining down on the small town of Newfield. The streets were bustling with people, and the air was filled with the sweet scent of flowers blooming in the gardens.

In the heart of the town, there was a quaint little cottage with a lush green garden. It was the home of a young painter named Lily, who had just moved to the town. She had always been fascinated by the vibrant colors of nature, and her art was a reflection of her love for it.

One day, as she was working on a painting in her garden, she heard a voice behind her.

"Excuse me, miss, but I couldn't help but notice your beautiful garden," said a gentleman who had just walked by.

Lily turned around to see a man who looked to be in his seventies. He had a kind face and a twinkle in his eye.

"Thank you, sir," replied Lily, "I love spending

time in my garden. It's my favorite place in the world."

The man smiled and said, "I know exactly what you mean. I used to have a garden just like this when I was young. It was my little piece of heaven on earth."

Lily was curious, so she asked him about his garden. The man's face lit up, and he started to tell her all about it.

"It was a beautiful garden, with roses of every color, lilies, and daisies. I used to spend hours tending to it, pruning the plants, and watering them. It was hard work, but it was worth it. The garden brought me so much joy and peace."

Lily listened to the man's story with interest. She could see the twinkle in his eye and the way his face lit up as he talked about his garden.

As they chatted, Lily realized that the man's love for his garden had never faded, even after all these years. She could see how much it still meant to him, and she knew that his memories of it would stay with him forever.

With a smile, Lily invited the man to come into

her garden and help her tend to it. The man eagerly accepted, and they spent the rest of the day working together, pruning the plants, watering them, and admiring the beauty of nature.

As the sun began to set, the man thanked Lily for the wonderful day.

"You know, young lady, you've reminded me of something today," he said with a smile.

"What's that?" asked Lily.

"That it's never too late to find joy in the things we love. Thank you for reminding me of that."

And with that, the man bid her farewell and walked away, leaving Lily alone in her garden.

As she sat there, basking in the warmth of the setting sun, Lily realized that the man had taught her a valuable lesson. She knew that no matter how old she got, she would always find joy in her garden and in the colors, sights, sounds, tastes, smells, and feelings of nature.

And with that, Lily picked up her paintbrush and started to work on a new painting. It was a painting of her garden, but it was more than that. It was a painting of the memories she had made that day, of the lesson she had learned, and of the joy she had found in the simple things in life.

The Sweet Scent of Memories

In the heart of a small town, nestled among the tall trees and rolling hills, lived an old woman named Mary. She was a woman of great character, with a warm smile and kind heart that drew people to her like bees to honey. She had lived a long life, filled with love, laughter, and the sweet scent of memories that lingered in her mind like the aroma of freshly baked cookies.

One day, as Mary was walking through the town square, she saw a young boy sitting alone on a bench. He looked sad and lost, with tears in his eyes and a heavy heart. Mary approached him and asked what was wrong.

The boy looked up at her with a pained expression and said, "My grandfather passed away yesterday, and I don't know how to deal with it. He was my best friend, my mentor, my everything."

Mary felt a pang of sympathy for the boy, knowing all too well the pain of losing someone you love. She sat down beside him and took his hand, offering him comfort and support.

As they sat together in silence, Mary began to share stories of her own life, of the people she had loved and lost, and the memories that kept them alive in her heart. She spoke of her grandmother's warm embrace, her father's hearty laughter, and the smell of her mother's cooking that always filled the house.

The boy listened intently, his tears drying as he was swept up in Mary's tales. He began to see the world through her eyes, filled with color, sights, sounds, tastes, smells, and feelings that stirred his soul and kept his imagination alive.

Mary's stories continued, each one more delightful and stimulating than the last. She spoke of the time she fell in love with a young man named John, and how he courted her with flowers and sweet words. She spoke of the day they married, surrounded by friends and family, and how they spent the rest of their lives together, filled with laughter, joy, and the sweet scent of memories.

As the sun began to set and the town square emptied, Mary and the boy remained on the bench, lost in their own thoughts and memories. They talked of life, of love, and of the beauty that surrounds us every day, if only we take the time to look for it.

Finally, as the stars began to twinkle in the night sky, the boy stood up and hugged Mary tightly. "Thank you," he said, his voice choked with emotion. "Thank you for sharing your memories with me. You've given me hope and comfort in a time of darkness."

Mary smiled warmly, her heart full of joy and contentment. "You're welcome, my dear," she said. "Remember, life is full of sweet scents and memories, and they will always be with you, even in the darkest of times."

As the boy walked away, his heart a little lighter and his spirit a little brighter, Mary sat alone on the bench, lost in her own thoughts and memories. She closed her eyes and breathed in the sweet scent of the night air, feeling grateful for the chance to share her stories and keep her memories alive.

The Comedy of Fate

On a cold winter's night in New York City, a young man named Jack found himself wandering the streets in search of warmth and shelter. He had lost his job and his apartment, and had nowhere to turn. As he walked aimlessly, shivering in the icy wind, he stumbled upon a small comedy club tucked away in an alleyway.

Curiosity piqued, Jack peered inside the club and was greeted by the sound of raucous laughter and applause. Without thinking, he slipped inside and found himself a seat at the back of the room.

Onstage, a comedian named Charlie was delivering a set that had the entire room in stitches. Jack had never laughed so hard in his life. For the first time in weeks, he forgot his troubles and felt alive again.

After the show, Jack approached Charlie and thanked him for the much-needed laughter. Charlie saw the sadness in Jack's eyes and took pity on him. "I have an idea," Charlie said. "I need a new writer for my act. Why don't you come work with me?"

Jack was skeptical but desperate, so he accepted the offer. Over the next few weeks, he and Charlie worked tirelessly on new material. They bounced ideas off each other and honed their delivery, perfecting the art of comedy.

Finally, the night of Charlie's big show arrived. The club was packed, and the atmosphere was electric. As they took the stage, Jack felt a sense of nervous excitement. He had never performed in front of so many people before.

They launched into their act, and the crowd roared with laughter. Jack couldn't believe it - they were killing it. He felt a sense of pride and accomplishment that he hadn't felt in years.

As they reached the climax of their set, Charlie suddenly turned to Jack and said, "I have a surprise for you." He pulled out an envelope and handed it to Jack. "This is for you. It's a check for all the hard work you've done. You deserve it."

Tears welled up in Jack's eyes as he opened the envelope. He couldn't believe it - the check was for ten thousand dollars. He had never seen so much money in his life.

After the show, Jack and Charlie walked out into

the chilly night air, both feeling euphoric. Suddenly, Charlie turned to Jack and said, "You know what, kid? You've got talent. You should keep doing this."

And that's exactly what Jack did. He became a successful comedian in his own right, thanks to Charlie's gift of laughter and the unexpected twist of fate that had brought them together.

Llife has a funny way of working out sometimes.